Diagnosis before First Aid

£7.95

Diagnosis before First Aid

A MANUAL FOR EMERGENCY CARE WORKERS

Neville Marsden M.R.C.S., L.R.C.P., D.Obst.R.C.O.G., Cert.Av.Med.

General Medical Practitioner; Clinical Assistant,
Orthopaedic Department, Burnley General Hospital.
Medical Officer to the Rossendale Fell Rescue Team.
Registrar for First Aid Examinations of the Medical
Subcommittee of the Mountain Rescue Committee
(England and Wales).

Foreword by

Noel F. Kirkman, M.D., F.R.C.S,
Honorary Consultant Surgeon at the University of
South Manchester; Chairman of the Mountain Rescue
Committee of England and Wales.

SECOND EDITION

CHURCHILL LIVINGSTONE
EDINBURGH LONDON MELBOURNE AND NEW YORK 1985

CHURCHILL LIVINGSTONE
Medical Division of Longman Group Limited

Distributed in the United States of America by
Churchill Livingstone Inc., 1560 Broadway, New York,
N.Y. 10036, and by associated companies, branches
and representatives throughout the world.

First edition 1978
Second edition 1985

ISBN 0-443-02837-0

British Library Cataloguing in Publication Data
Marsden, Neville
    Diagnosis before first aid: a manual for
    emergency care workers.—2nd ed.
    1. First aid in illness and injury
    2. Diagnosis
    I. Title
    616.02'52   RC87

Library of Congress Cataloging in Publication Data
Marsden, Neville.
    Diagnosis before first aid.
    Includes bibliographies and index.
    1. First aid in illness and injury.   2. Diagnosis.
I. Title. [DNLM: 1. Allied Health Personnel.
2. Diagnosis.   3. First Aid.   WA 292 M364d]
RC86.7.M37   1985   616.02'4   84-21419

Produced by Longman Singapore Publishers (Pte) Ltd.
Printed in Singapore.

Foreword

Despite the variety of first aid manuals available, this book fills a vacant niche because of its fresh and occasionally unorthodox style and the insistence of as good a diagnosis as possible in the field. This emphasis on diagnosis as a prerequisite for satisfactory first aid is highly commendable.

Dr Neville Marsden's exposition of the head to toe examination of casualties in a systematic way and his recurrent reiteration of the importance of comparing the injured to the uninjured part or side will be fully supported by all who teach first aid or work in a casualty department. The clear illustrations effectively emphasise many of the points made in the text. The first aider may perhaps save a life on some rare occasion if he has read and remembered the account of tracheotomy. Dr Marsden justly stresses the need to make every available effort to dislodge the foreign body obstructing the larynx before this heroic procedure is attempted.

This book is the outcome of many first aid courses which Dr Marsden has given to mountain rescue team members and other emergency care workers; it has been prompted by their problems and questions.

Although primarily written for the active first aider, this book could be read with profit by physiotherapists and medical students in the early years of their courses. It is a welcome addition to the literature on the constantly growing problems of first aid.

1977   Noel F. Kirkman

Preface to the Second Edition

In this edition, some modifications have been made to the original text in order to clarify certain points. In particular, 'Exposure' has been expanded considerably to include the effects of heat and altitude, as well as to distinguish between one type of hypothermia and the others. A number of additions to the text have been made, notably 'Adder bite', 'Anaphylactic shock', 'The classical stages of anaesthesia', 'The shunting sign' (another early sign of death), 'Principles of treatment of fractures', 'Burns', 'Summary of injury and non-injury conditions of the chest', 'Summary of injury and non-injury conditions of the abdomen' and 'The search for injuries in the unconscious patient.'. The contents of this book should now cover, more than adequately, the First Aid syllabus of the Mountain Rescue Committee of England and Wales and, I would hope, many other first aid syllabuses.

The aforementioned modifications and additions have been prompted, yet again, by (on the one hand) First Aiders and (on the other hand) by my own search for ways to explain certain matters to my students during First Aid courses. I value the stimulus of my continued involvement in the teaching of First Aid.

I am very grateful to my friend, Mr Norman Astbury, for his most able assistance with additional art work in this edition, and also to Mrs Geraldine Hope and Mrs Karen Stevens for their work on the typescript. Finally, my thanks are due, once again, to Mrs Mary Emmerson Law of Churchill Livingstone, whose patience, I trust, has been rewarded at last.

Lancashire, 1985   N. M.

Preface to the First Edition

Over a period of a few years, I have met First Aiders belonging to various organisations. I suppose that this was more or less inevitable since I have been a full-time casualty officer. I am now a part-time casualty officer, my main occupation being General Practice.

The first thing about First Aiders which impresses me, is their obvious enthusiasm for First Aid. The second thing which impresses me, is their desire to increase their own knowledge and ability.

It was their thirst for knowledge which prompted me to write this book. I would not have known what to write without first finding out what the First Aiders wanted and needed to know, and I found this out through personal contact with them. I hope that I have provided the answers to their questions.

For their reading and constructive criticism of the manuscript I wish to express my thanks to Peter Durst, Leader of the Rossendale Fell Rescue Team, to Corporal Trevor Loftus, Deputy Leader of the R.A.F. (Stafford) Mountain Rescue Team, and last, but by no means least, to Dr A. S. G. ('Tony') Jones, Leader of the Ogwen Valley Mountain Rescue Team in North Wales. By their comments and suggestions, all three have made valuable contributions to this book. I am further indebted to Trevor Loftus for all the diagrams and cartoons, and also to Henry Stott, Brian Veevers and Bryan Wilson (members of the Rossendale Fell Rescue Team), who helped a great deal towards the production of the diagrams of limb movements. I wish to thank Mrs Susan M. Dunning for typing the manuscript, and also the publishers, Churchill Livingstone, for their co-operation. Finally, for his foreword, I thank Mr Noel F. Kirkman; I am proud to count myself amongst his former students.

Lancashire, 1977   N. M.

Contents

Contents

Introduction

This book is based on a series of talks given to the Rossendale Fell Rescue Team. The text is written in such a way as to give the impression that the author is speaking in person to the reader. This should make for easy reading of the text.

The objects of this book are to improve the First Aider's ability to diagnose and to improve the First Aider's understanding of the injured person. If a First Aider can achieve these two objectives, then he, or she, will be far more competent than before when dealing with the single casualty, and will also be better able to decide correctly on the order of priority for evacuation when dealing with mass casualties. Therefore, in order to concentrate attention on diagnosis, a great deal about treatment has been omitted purposely. Treatment is quite adequately dealth with in numerous books on First Aid. However, treatment varies from time to time whereas diagnosis does not. A fractured clavicle is a fractured clavicle whether it is treated by broad-arm sling or by a figure-of-eight bandage.

First Aiders tend to concentrate on practising First Aid treatment such as splinting, bandaging and mouth-to-mouth respiration. This is *not* the logical approach to First Aid. *Diagnosis must always precede treatment.* Some injuries are obvious but others are not. This book will teach the First Aider to search for those injuries which are not obvious. As he, or she, reads this book and *practises* what he, or she, is told to practise, it will become evident to the First Aider that the logical approach to any injured person is history, examination, diagnosis and *then* treatment.

The book is divided into Parts I, II and III. Please read them in that order. Part I is necessarily factual, and facts tend to be boring. However, it is essential to read Part I thoroughly if Parts II and III are to be understood properly. I have tried to include only the essential facts, without producing a whole textbook on human biology. Part II deals with History and Examination and, in particular, with the system of head-to-toe examination which the First Aider is encouraged to practise as much as possible. It is an efficient method of examination. It saves time, eliminates doubt, and therefore increases the First Aider's confidence. Part III deals with specific subjects.

I trust that the First Aider will enjoy this book, and that after reading it and practising what is preached, his, or her, diagnostic ability and understanding of the injured person will have improved considerably.

PART I

How do we function?

1

Basic functions

Diagnosis depends on our ability to recognise the abnormal. If we are to recognise the abnormal, then it is logical that we should first learn to know what is normal. Therefore, it is necessary to have a basic understanding of the normal functions of the human body before we proceed any further. In fact, it is so necessary, that medical students spend two years learning about the normal human body before they even begin to learn about illness and injury.

Basically, the human body is a living mechanism which needs energy for its function and survival. Energy is obtained by the combination of food products with oxygen in the tissues. The food products are obtained from the food we eat, and oxygen is obtained via the lungs. Both oxygen and the food products are transported to the tissues by the bloodstream, which also carries away the waste products of energy production from the tissues. These waste products are excreted via the lungs and kidneys. The food residue, which is the unuseable part of the food we eat, is eliminated as faeces.

The cell

This is the basic unit of the body. We are composed of millions upon millions of cells, which are so small that they can be seen only with the aid of a microscope. There are many different types of cell. It is not necessary for the First Aider to know them all. It is sufficient to say that each cell of the body has its own particular function to perform and it is constructed appropriately. For example, the red and white cells of the blood are rounded to facilitate travel within the bloodstream, whereas the cells which form the inner linings of the blood vessels are very thin, flat and smooth to prevent turbulent blood flow, which could lead to the formation of a blood clot. Muscle cells can vary their length; they can contract or relax. On the other hand, nerve cells cannot vary their length.

They transmit nerve impulses from one part of the body to another. A nerve cell may be very long indeed but if it is stretched it will be damaged. So, every cell has its own special function to perform and it contributes to the function of the human body as a whole.

The alimentary system

The word 'alimentary' simply means the mouth, throat, gullet, stomach, small intestine, large intestine, rectum and anus, in that order. It is the food-tube which passes right through us from one end to the other. Food is chewed in the mouth and swallowed down the gullet into the stomach, where it is churned up by the muscular action of the stomach and partly broken down by the stomach's acid juice. From the stomach the food is passed into the small intestine, where a number of chemical juices break it down into its basic components, *viz*:

1. Carbohydrates—i.e. sugars, e.g. from bread and potatoes.
2. Fatty acids—these are the basic components of fats.
3. Amino acids—Sorry, but there is no other name for these. Amino acids are the basic chemical 'bricks' used to build up proteins.

When the food has been broken down into these food products, it is passed along the bowel by rhythmic bowel movements, and these movements give rise to *bowel sounds*, which can be heard by placing your ear to someone else's abdomen. *Try it.* You will need to listen for bowel sounds later, when you come to examine the abdomen, so you may as well get used to recognising normal bowel sounds *now*!

Eventually, the food products are absorbed through the bowel wall, and they are taken, via the bloodstream and the lymphatic vessels, to the liver for storage. From the liver, the sugars can be sent (as glucose) to the muscles, via the bloodstream, to be used for energy production. The amino acids can be sent to any part of the body to be build up into new proteins, which will replace old, worn-out proteins. The fats are stored all over the body in fat depots. A very important fat depot is the fat deposited under the skin. This helps to insulate the body against the cold. Fats are also a reserve supply of energy, although energy can be obtained much more rapidly from glucose.

The unwanted by-products of digestion are known as the food residue. This is passed into the large bowel, where as much water as possible is absorbed from it. This is one of the body's *fluid-*

conservation mechanisms. (These mechanisms are important and will be referred to again.) The remainder of the food residue is passed out through the anus at intervals as faeces (i.e. 'stools').

The above is a very brief description of the function of the human digestive system. Just how brief it is can be judged by the fact that research workers can spend a whole lifetime studying it. Let us now consider the body's use of the sugars, etc., which it has acquired from plants or from other animals.

Metabolism

Metabolism is simply a word which, in a nutshell, means, 'The production and use of energy'. Thus, we can use one word instead of six; it saves time, and besides that, later on, I shall refer to something called the metabolic rate. (The metabolic rate is the *rate* of production and use of energy). We use energy for all our activities, and one very important activity is to maintain our body temperatures at the correct level of 37°C (98.6°F), or slightly below this. If our body temperature falls to 25°C (77°F), we are well and truly in a state of hypothermia, and if it falls to 20°C (68°F) we will die. So, in order to stay alive and healthy, we must maintain a body temperature of 37°C (98.6°F). Our muscles use energy when we move about, or even when we stand still, because in standing still, our muscle-actions are balancing each other, so that we do not fall over. The heart uses energy to pump blood around the circulatory system. In fact, every cell which goes to make up the human body uses energy, and in order to produce energy the following processes may occur:

1. Glucose reacts with oxygen to produce water, carbon dioxide and energy.
2. Fats can be broken down slowly to produce water, carbon dioxide and energy.
3. Proteins can be broken down to give urea, water, carbon dioxide and energy.

The exact methods by which these processes occur are very complicated indeed, but it is not necessary for you to know exactly how they work. It is quite sufficient for you to know that these three mechanisms of energy-production exist.

The metabolic rate varies according to age, build and sex. Babies have a high metabolic rate, because they have to grow from about 7 lb (3.55 kg) at birth to about 28 lb (14.2 kg) at the age of twelve months. Babies are particularly vulnerable to hypothermia, because

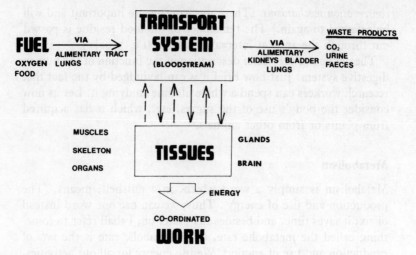

Fig. 1

they can burn up their energy reserves very rapidly. Therefore, babies have to be well clothed, to prevent excessive heat loss, and they have to be fed more times per day than adults in order to keep up their energy supplies. A young baby's main occupation is sleeping, because the baby's energy is largely devoted to multiplying its cells, in order to grow bigger. As the infant grows into a child, the metabolic rate begins to decrease slightly. Height increases by spurts of growth, which occur about every two years. The growth in height by girls usually precedes that of boys until late teenage life, when the boys put on a final spurt to become taller than the girls, on average. As a rule, a girl matures sexually about two years ahead of a boy of her own age.

We reach our physical peak at about twenty-eight years of age, after which we begin the *ageing process*. Our metabolic rate decreases gradually, together with a very gradual decline in our physical and mental prowess and our ability to regenerate and repair any damage to our bodies, i.e. wounds and fractures take longer to heal. The difference in metabolic rate between a man of forty years and a man of twenty years explains why the younger man with a higher metabolic rate, is likely to develop hypothermia sooner than the older man with the lower metabolic rate, who is better able to conserve his energy. Likewise a slim young girl would develop hypothermia faster than an older fatter woman. In general, women can resist hypothermia better than men do because:

a. they tend to have a lower metabolic rate, and

b. they have a thicker layer of fat underneath the skin, which gives them better insulation against the cold, than men have.

We shall consider metabolism further in Chapter 8 when discussing Hypothermia, under the sub-heading, 'Exposure.'

Excretion and kidney function

Excretion is the process by which the unwanted by-products of metabolism are eliminated from the body, i.e. excess water, excess carbon dioxide and urea. *Carbon dioxide*, produced by cell metabolism, passes into the blood, which transports it to the lungs from where it is passed out of the body with the expired air. However, carbon dioxide, when dissolved in water forms a bicarbonate ion, which can be excreted by the kidneys *selectively*. The kidneys can regulate the amount of bicarbonate ions excreted, and this is important in maintaining the correct pH of the body. (This will be explained later.) *Urea* is a completely harmless by-product of protein metabolism and it is of no further use to the body. Therefore, the kidneys simply excrete it as it reaches them, via the bloodstream. *Water* is a very necessary substance for our existence. In fact, about 60 per cent of our total body weight is water. It is possible for a human being to survive for about one month on fresh water alone and no food; but without water we can survive only a few days. Even so, it is necessary to have the right amount of water in us, and any excess is excreted by the kidneys. Water can also be lost by sweating, and as water vapour (small amounts) in the expired air.

The kidneys perform their functions by acting as elaborate filtering mechanisms. About one fifth of the blood pumped out by the heart in any given minute passes through the kidneys. As the blood passes through the kidneys, a fair volume of the plasma is filtered into tiny tubes. These tiny tubes (or tubules) reabsorb water, glucose and the minerals, etc., required by the body, whilst at the same time not reabsorbing urea. The tubules are highly selective in their ability to reabsorb (or not to reabsorb) the chemical substances which filter through to them, and are therefore able to regulate the chemical balance of the body fluids. For the chemically minded First Aiders, the body fluids must be kept slightly alkaline; i.e. they must be kept within a range of pH of 7.2–7.6 (average pH 7.4). Any variation outside this range is *lethal* to human beings.

For the non-chemically minded First Aiders, I should explain that pH is a term used to describe acidity or alkalinity, e.g. pH 1.0 means that a substance is very strongly acid; pH 12.0 means that a substance is very strongly alkaline and pH 7.0 is neutral.

The kidney functions, therefore, are extremely delicate and complicated, but they can be summarised briefly as follows:
1. Excretion of urea (and other substances no longer required).
2. Reabsorption of glucose (and other substances required).
3. Regulation of pH.
4. Regulation of chemical composition of body fluids.
5. Reabsorption of water, i.e. *fluid conservation* (except for the amount of water necessary to form urine).

Once the urine is formed, it passes from the kidneys, down the ureters to the bladder, where it is stored. At intervals, the bladder is emptied by passing the urine to the outside world, via the urethra.

Circulation, respiration and blood pressure

The heart is the strong muscular pump which pushes the blood round the whole circulatory system. Blood is pumped through the lungs, where carbon dioxide passes out of the blood into the air sacs of the lungs. At the same time, oxygen passes from the air sacs of the lungs into the blood. In fact, it is the haemoglobin inside the red cells of the blood, which carries carbon dioxide to the lungs and oxygen away from the lungs. The oxygen is acquired by inhaling and the carbon dioxide is expelled by exhaling. When the blood reaches the tissues the reverse happens—the red cells give up their oxygen, which passes into the tissue cells, and the tissue cells give up carbon dioxide, which passes into the red cells. This whole process is called *respiration*.

After passing through the lungs, the blood returns to the heart and it is then distributed to the rest of the body via the aorta. The aorta gives off smaller arteries, which in turn give off even smaller arteries, until a system of tiny vessels called *arterioles* is reached. The arteries have *elastic* walls, and are therefore capable of expansion and recoil (it is the expansion of the radial artery, for example, which you can feel in the pulse at the wrist). The arterioles, however, are important little blood vessels, because they have *muscular* walls. This enables them to control the flow of blood through them, because each arteriole can alter its calibre. If an arteriole constricts, it will reduce the amount of blood passing through it, but if it dilates (by relaxing its muscular wall), it will increase the amount of blood flowing through it. *Therefore, the amount of blood-flow to any part of the body at any particular time is determined by the state of constriction, or dilation, of the arterioles in that part of the body at that particular time.* This is a very important fact. When we are at rest after a meal, the arterioles controlling blood supply to the gut open up, because our digestive processes are at work, but the arterioles to our muscles tend to shut down, because we are resting. When we are running, working etc., the reverse occurs. In other words, our arterioles enable us to send blood to the places which most need it at any given time.

After passing through the arterioles the blood enters a system of microscopic vessels in the tissues called *capillaries*, and it is here that the cells exchange carbon dioxide for a fresh supply of oxygen. The blood then enters a system of minute *venules*, which merge to form *veins*, which in turn, merge to form larger veins until the blood finally reaches the heart via the vena cava, and the whole process is repeated.

Blood pressure

As the heart pushes blood around the circulatory system, the blood is under a certain amount of pressure. If the blood was not under any pressure at all, then it would not move, would it? When the heart contracts (i.e. pumps), we call the period of contraction *systole*, and the period during which the heart relaxes is called *diastole*. So, when the heart pumps blood out into the aorta, the blood pressure rises to a peak which is known as the *systolic blood pressure*. When the heart relaxes, the blood pressure falls to a basic level, called the *diastolic blood pressure*.

A typical systolic blood pressure would be 120 mmHg, and a typical diastolic blood pressure would be 70 mmHg. This would be recorded as, 'B.P. — $\frac{120}{70}$'. The blood pressure varies from one individual to another, but the accepted normal maximum readings are 140 mmHg for the systolic and 90 mmHg for the diastolic blood pressure. The instrument used to measure blood pressure is called a sphygmomanometer (or 'sphyg.' for brevity). A description of the sphygmomanometer and how to use it will be given in Section II.

Before we leave this topic, I will clarify what is meant by the term *Pulse Pressure*. This is simply the difference between the systolic and diastolic blood pressures. So, take away the diastolic from the systolic blood pressure and you have the pulse pressure, e.g.:

1. B.P. $= \frac{120}{70}$ Therefore, pulse pressure $= 120-70 = 50$ mmHg
2. B.P. $= \frac{140}{80}$ Therefore, pulse pressure $= 140-80 = 60$ mmHg

Incidentally, the blood pressure is *usually* measured in terms of millimeters of mercury (mmHg). Some people measure the blood pressure in dynes.

The adrenal glands

These are two small, pyramid-shaped glands which lie above the kidneys (one adrenal gland above each kidney). For this reason, they are sometimes called the suprarenal glands ('supra' = above; 'renal' = appertaining to the kidney). Each gland consists of a central part called the medulla, which produces a chemical substance called epinephrine. This is a mixture of adrenaline and noradrenaline. The outer part of the gland is called the cortex, and this produces Cortisone and other related chemicals.

During exercise, epinephrine is released into the circulation. It causes an increase in heart rate and pulse pressure and in the rate at which the blood circulates, because extra supplies of glucose and oxygen are needed by the muscles. If we are startled, or injured, adrenaline is suddenly injected into the circulation by the adrenal glands, and this causes a sudden increase in heart rate. This explains why you can feel your heart pounding when you are startled or frightened. In fact, a good way to remember the effects of the *adrenaline response* as it is called, is to say that it prepares us for *Fright, Fight and Flight*. Another effect of the adrenaline response is to reduce our ability to feel pain. This is just as important as it is logical. For instance, if an animal is injured in a fight, is losing the fight, and decides that there is no future in continuing the fight, then it breaks off the engagement and runs away. This is 'Flight', and obviously, during its flight for safety, it does not wish its ability to run to be impaired by pain. Adrenaline provides this lowered pain sensibility. The animal feels the pain later, when it has reached safety, and when the adrenaline response has worn off. Exactly the same response occurs in human beings, and it is important to remember this, because a fracture may remain painless for a few hours after injury, as a result of the adrenaline response. I remember well a man who had broken both wrists in a car crash.

His face was pale because of the adrenaline response (i.e. 'Fright') and he could not use his hands because of the fractures, but he felt no pain. Even by moving the fractures so that I caused bony crepitus (see *Injuries to Bones and Joints*), I could not cause him to feel pain. It was only six hours after the injury, when the adrenaline response wore off, that he began to feel any pain at all!

2

Fluids and fluid conservation

The blood

Basically, blood is a fluid composed of water, minerals, glucose, proteins, red blood cells and white blood cells. If we remove the red and white cells from the blood, the remaining fluid is plasma. Plasma is a very useful substance, because it can be dried and converted into a solid, just as milk can be converted to powder. When a patient reaches hospital and needs an urgent transfusion of blood, a sample of his blood must be sent to the laboratory for cross-matching with the blood which is to be given to him. This is to ensure that his blood will not clot the red cells of the blood transfused into him. If that happened, the results would be disastrous. The cross-matching of blood can take up to one and a half hours, and this could be too long a delay for the patient. This is where the dried plasma can play a great role. By mixing the dried plasma with sterile water, the plasma becomes fluid again. It does not have to be cross-matched, can be given to the patient straight away and results in a marked improvement in the patient's general condition. Dried plasma can be stored for years and is reconstituted in two minutes.

The functions of the various constituents of the blood are as follows:

1. *Red cells*. These carry oxygen from the lungs to the tissues, and carbon dioxide from the tissues to the lungs.

2. *White cells*. These fight invading bacteria, and have certain other functions.

3. *Proteins*. These have three basic functions:

a. Clotting. A whole series of proteins take part in the clotting mechanism, which is very complex indeed.

b. Antibodies. These are the proteins which neutralise the poisons produced by bacteria.

c. Viscosity of the blood, i.e. the proteins help to keep the blood at its correct 'stickiness'. They stop it from becoming too watery.

4. *Chemical substances*. The main chemical substances in the blood are sodium ions, potassium ions, chloride ions and bicarbonate ions. The relative concentrations of these ions are delicately balanced in order to maintain the correct pH of the body (see *Kidney Function*, pp. 7 and 8).

5. *Water*. This is the constituent which keeps the blood fluid.

The skin

The skin is divided basically into two main layers, the epidermis and the dermis.

1. *The epidermis*. This is the outside, or superficial layer. It has about five layers of cells. The deepest layer of cells is called the germinal layer. It produces cells which are pushed towards the surface. As the cells approach the surface they die, become flattened and eventually they flake off. This flattened, dead layer of cells forms a barrier, which is impervious to water. In other words, we have found yet another *fluid-conservation mechanism*. In fact, but for this water-impervious layer in our skins, we would all walk around dripping fluid at such a rate that we would no be able to drink water fast enough to replace the fluid lost!

2. *The dermis*. This is the deeper layer of the skin. Unlike the epidermis, it has a good supply of blood vessels. It also has hair follicles, from which hairs grow out beyond the skin surface. The sweat glands also originate in the dermis, as do the sebaceous glands, which secrete an oily substance onto the surface of the skin. Beneath the dermis there is a layer of fat.

Let us summarise the functions of the skin:

a. If offers a certain amount of protection to underlying structures.

b. It conserves fluid.

c. It produces sebaceous fluid which:
   (i) helps to stop the skin from drying up;
   (ii) discourages unwanted bacteria from inhabiting the skin because it is alkaline;
   (iii) lubricates the bases of the hairs, so that they bend rather than break.

d. *Temperature regulation*. This is a very important function. When the body is becoming over-heated, the blood vessels in the dermis dilate. This increases the blood-flow near the surface of the body. Since blood is warm, this means that there is more heat available for direct radiation to the surface of the body and then away to the atmosphere. If this does not get rid of enough excess heat, then the sweat glands come into operation. They secrete a film of very dilute salt solution (sweat) onto the surface of the skin. When the film of sweat evaporates from the body surface, then (in accordance with the laws of physics) heat is lost from the body surface.

When the temperature of our surroundings falls below a certain level, the blood vessels in the dermis reduce heat loss to a minimum by constricting themselves and reducing the blood-flow through the dermis to a minute quantity. However, this constriction of blood vessels in the dermis cannot last indefinitely, otherwise the skin itself would die from lack of nourishment. So, eventually the vessels in the dermis must re-dilate, and when they do so, they over-dilate in order to compensate for the time during which the skin has been relatively undernourished. This compensatory over-dilation is called *reactive hyperaemia*—just think of how pink your fingers become when you warm your hands in front of the fire, after being out on a cold winter's day! Now, this reactive hyperaemia is perfectly natural and safe, *provided* that we have found a place of shelter and warmth. However, if someone becomes extremely deeply hypothermic, without finding shelter, and if his skin vessels cannot constrict any longer, then reactive hyperaemia will occur, giving him the sensation of a warm glow all over, but he will die quickly, owing to the rapid heat-loss which will ensue.

Body fluids

I have made mention of fluid-conservation mechanisms already. Let us now list the organs involved in fluid-conservation. They are:
1. The skin (impervious to water).
2. The kidneys (they lose only as much water as is necessary to form urine).
3. The large bowel (it absorbs as much fluid as possible from the food residue).

If the kidneys or the large bowel are malfunctioning then there is nothing much that the First Aider can do about it. However, I would like to stress at this point, that *a great deal of fluid can be lost from a superficial burn*, i.e. from a burn which has destroyed only the superficial, water-impervious layer of the skin, leaving the dermis intact. I have actually seen half a pint of plasma drip from a superficial burn on a man's forearm in a matter of only ten minutes. At that rate, he would have lost three pints of fluid in one hour! The treatment of this kind of burn is to cover up the burn (as instructed in the First Aid Manuals) and to cover the dressing with a good, *firm* bandage. The principle involved here is that the pressure of the bandage should exceed the pressure under which the plasma is oozing through the surface of the burn, and this should reduce fluid loss to a minimum.

Let us now turn our attention to the distribution of the body fluids. As stated before, about 60 per cent of the human body is composed of fluid. Most of this fluid is inside the cells and is known as Intracellular Fluid (ICF). All the fluid which is outside the cells is known as Extracellular Fluid (ECF). From a strictly technical viewpoint, ECF includes blood, since blood is outside the tissue cells. From a purely practical point of view, it is better to regard blood as a separate fluid from the rest of the ECF. So, in this book, whenever the term 'ECF' is used, it will refer to all of the extra-cellular fluid, excluding the blood. The reason for this will soon become apparent.

In general, women have slightly less fluid per kilogram of body weight than men. The body fluids of a man who weighs 70 kg (11 stones) can be summarised as follows:

		Litres	*Pints* (approx.)
Total blood volume	=	4.92	$8\frac{1}{2}$
ECF (excluding blood)	=	6.08	$10\frac{1}{2}$
ICF	=	32.00	$56\frac{1}{2}$
Total body fluids	=	43.00	$75\frac{1}{2}$

The practical importance of ECF

It is the human equivalent of the hump on the camel's back. In other words, it is a valuable reserve of fluid for emergencies. This applies particularly when blood is lost. Reserves of fluid can be drawn from the ECF, via the capillaries, into the blood vessels in order to make up for the volume of blood lost, although ECF can never make up for the loss of red cells. This ability to replenish blood volume after blood loss, prevents the heart from going into failure (which would happen if the blood volume continued to decline). So, it can be appreciated that if this store of ECF did not exist, then many people would not live long enough after injury to reach hospital and be transfused. In fact, many people, now alive after injury, would be dead. These people owe their lives to *blood transfusion*, because the only real replacement for blood is blood.

The existence of ECF, and its function during emergencies, cre-ates a valuable time interval for casualties after injury. Please re-

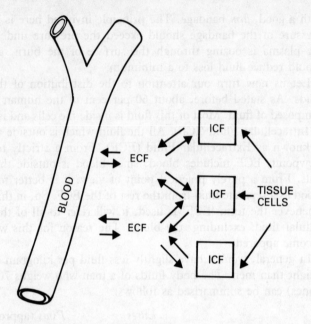

Fig. 2 Interrelationship of blood, ECF and ICF

member that *THIS TIME IS VALUABLE*, and it should never be wasted. There is a limit to the amount of ECF which can be drawn into the bloodstream, and there is a limit to the number of red cells which the casualty can afford to lose. So, if an injured person needs blood, secure the airway, stop haemorrhage, spend no more time than is absolutely necessary on splinting and get him as quickly as possible to the place where blood is available—HOSPITAL!

If the journey to hospital is likely to be protracted, an intravenous drip can be of tremendous (indeed life-saving) value, by boosting the circulating blood volume and, therefore, avoiding depletion of ECF and ICF. Plasma, dextrose, saline and synthetic solutions of low-molecular-weight proteins (often referred to as 'plasma expanders') are all useful. However, in the U.K. at the present time, the laws prohibit first aiders from introducing a needle into a vein for any purpose, since only medically qualified personnel are allowed to perform intravenous techniques. In other countries (notably the U.S.A.), paramedical personnel are trained in intravenous techniques.

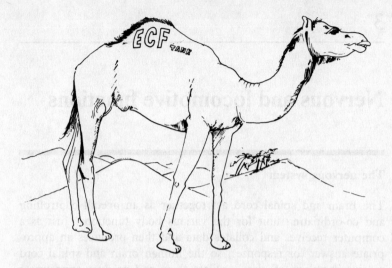

Fig. 3 'ECF is the human equivalent of the hump on the camel's back.'

The lymphatic system

This was mentioned briefly before in connection with the absorption of fats from the intestine. In fact, it is basically a separate vascular system, which collects excess ECF and takes it back slowly to rejoin the main bloodstream. It is also rich in white cells and lymph nodes, both of which are concerned with the defence against bacteria.

The spleen

The entire functions of this organ are still not known. We do know that it contains a reserve supply of red cells, which it can inject into the circulation in an emergency, e.g. sudden heavy blood loss. Otherwise, as far as the First Aider is concerned, the spleen exists in order to be injured!

3

Nervous and locomotive functions

The nervous system

The brain and spinal cord act together as an overall controlling and co-ordinating unit for the various body functions. Just as a computer receives and collates data and then produces an appropriate answer (or response), so the human brain and spinal cord receive impulses (cf. data), collate them and produce appropriate responses.

You do not need a detailed knowledge of this. *Sensory impulses*, e.g. touch, pain, pressure – from all parts of the body (skin, muscles, joints etc.) travel along the nerves towards the spinal cord and then up the spinal cord to the brain. *Motor impulses* originating in the brain (and usually triggered off by the arrival of a sensory impulse) travel down the spinal cord and out along the nerves to the muscles, which, being stimulated by the motor impulse, then contract. This is a very simple explanation of the basic way in which the nervous system works.

Some impulses reach conscious level (e.g. pain), but there are many which do not. For example, when you are standing, you are aware that you are standing but you are not aware of the hundreds of nervous impulses shooting up and down the spinal cord in order to keep you standing. The same applies to walking. When you wish to walk, you walk; but what you are not aware of is the fact that every step involves hundreds of nervous impulses, and muscle and joint movements. If we had to initiate from *conscious* level every nervous impulse necessary to enable us to walk, then life would be very slow and difficult indeed!

Likewise, blood-flow to certain areas at certain times, heart rate and respiratory rate are controlled by nervous impulses, over which the vast majority of people have no voluntary control at all. (Some people can slow, or even stop, their own hearts at will—i.e. voluntarily – but such people are extremely rare individuals.)

There are two other important factors which I should mention. The first is, that the right side of the cerebrum (brain) controls the movements of the left side of the body, and vice versa. This is useful to remember when dealing with someone who has had a stroke. The second important factor is that the *speech centre* in right-handed people is in the left cerebrum. In left-handed people it is in the right cerebrum. Therefore, if a right-handed person has a stroke in the right cerebrum, causing paralysis in the left arm and leg, then he will still be able to speak, although his speech may be affected by weakness of the left side of the face. If a right-handed person has a stroke in the left cerebrum (affecting the right arm and leg), then he will almost certainly lose his ability to speak coherently, because the speech centre is almost invariably affected. For a left-handed person, the situations are reversed.

The bones

The bones of a living person are *alive*. They maintain our shape by giving support to the softer tissues. The basic component of bone is a protein called *ossein*, and this protein is formed into the structure of each individual bone by bone-forming cells called *osteoblasts*. Calcium salts are deposited in the ossein in order to add rigidity to the bone. Old and damaged bone is removed by cells and *osteoclasts*, which thus make way for the osteoblasts to move in and lay down new bone. This process of renewal of bone goes on constantly throughout our lives. If it did not occur, then spontaneous fractures would occur when bones had been in use for a certain length of time, just as fatigue fractures can occur in metals, which have been in service for a long time.

Since bone is a living substance, every bone has a blood supply of its own. Therefore, when a bone is broken, the vessels in it are torn and blood can then flow out of the bone fragments at the fracture site. This is an important fact. *Broken bones bleed*, and the amount of blood lost depends on which bone is broken. In general, the larger the bone, the greater the blood loss. Since the blood vessels in bones are relatively small, the blood is lost at a fairly slow rate, usually over a period of three hours or more; but the blood is lost from the circulation, just as surely as if it had poured out onto the ground. To maintain its function as a transport mechanism for oxygen, carbon dioxide, etc., blood must move around within the vascular system. The estimate of blood loss from various bones is dealt with in Section III (*Injuries to Bones and Joints*).

Joints

There are different types of joint in the body, but those with which you are principally concerned are the joints of the limbs, and these are synovial joints. A synovial joint is formed between the ends of two or more bones. The bone ends are covered with a special kind of cartilage, called articular cartilage, which allows the bone ends to move smoothly against each other. The joint is surrounded by a tough capsule, inside which there is a delicate lining called the synovium. The synovium produces an oily fluid, called synovial fluid, which lubricates the joint.

The muscles

Muscles are composed of cells which can vary their length. When a muscle shortens (i.e. contracts) then the parts of the bones to which the muscle is attached, are brought closer to each other. In this way, the position of the joint between the two bones is altered. When the muscle relaxes, the joint is allowed to move the other way. Muscles are usually arranged in groups which work opposite each other, e.g. one group of muscles bends the elbow and the other group extends the elbow.

Having summarised the normal functions of the body, we can now start to learn how to diagnose the abnormal.

History and examination

4

The history

When a doctor approaches a patient, the first thing he does is to ask questions. This is known, in the medical fraternity, as taking the history. The history can be divided into 'present' and 'previous' histories.

A. Present history

From a First Aider's point of view, the present history will almost always be concerned with an injury. Therefore, the following questions will be asked:

1. 'What happened?'
2. 'How did it happen?'
3. 'Where does it hurt?' (This gives a clue to the site or sites of injury.)
4. 'Have you been unconscious?' or 'Were you knocked out?'
5. 'Can you move your limbs and wiggle your toes?' (especially important when neck or back injury is suspected).

The above questions are a reasonable guide-line, but a word of caution to you. If somebody says, 'I fell,' then that is not enough. You must ask the following two questions: 'How far did you fall?' and 'How did you land?' There are two reasons for these two questions. Firstly, the farther a person falls, the worse his injuries are likely to be. Secondly, the part of the body which makes contact with the ground first is the part most likely to be injured. Having said that, I must state that it is common knowledge amongst orthopaedic surgeons (the 'bone and joint' surgeons) that if a man falls about twenty feet and lands on one or both feet, then, although the heels and ankles are the parts most likely to suffer, the force of the impact with the ground is transmitted upwards through the lower limbs to the pelvis and then continues up the spine to the base of the skull. It is therefore important to remember that, if a man falls twenty feet or more and lands on his feet, he may sustain fractures

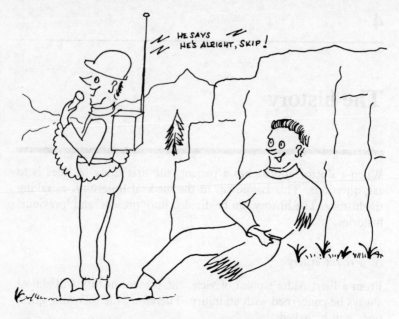

Fig. 4 Never simply accept the patient's word that he's alright.

in any of the bones of the lower limbs, in the pelvis, the spinal bones or even in the base of the skull. This is a very important lesson to learn. So, remember the saying: 'The words, "I fell", should ring a bell.' This will remind you to ask how far the man fell and how he landed.

Question 4, 'Have you been unconscious?', is important, because in my experience, many people will not volunteer the fact that they have been unconscious. Perhaps they think that I know already, or perhaps they think that it does not matter now because they have recovered consciousness. Sometimes a person may not realise that he has been unconscious, in which case, the evidence of witnesses of the injury can be valuable. In any case, I always ask the question, just to make sure. Preferably, ask any witnesses *first* and then ask the patient. You will realise the importance of this when you read *Head Injuries*, in Part III.

B. Previous history

This can be of great importance. For example, if a person is unconscious and a friend is with him, it would be useful to know if the

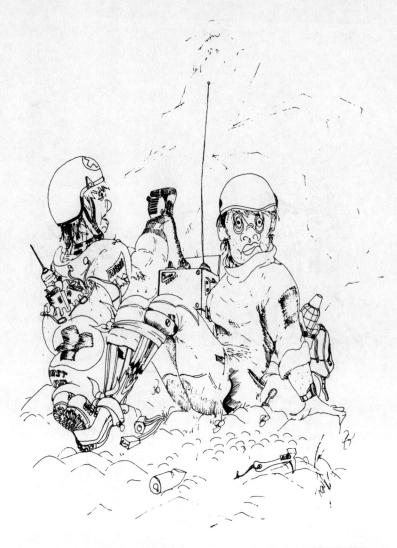

Fig. 5 Check the casualty's history.

unconscious man is a known diabetic or epileptic. Similarly, if a man has had his right kidney removed at some time in the past, it would be foolish to make a diagnosis of rupture, or suspected rupture, of the right kidney in his case!

I have found that the least time-consuming approach to the previous history is to ask the following questions in this order:

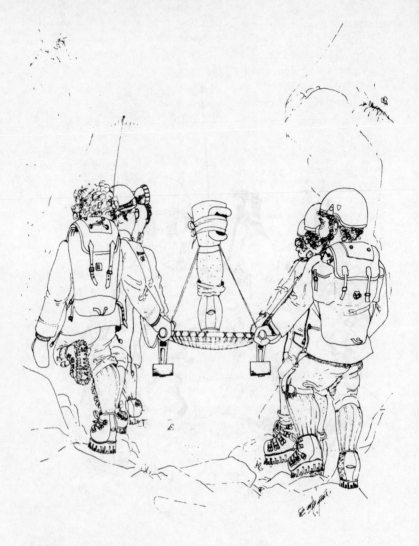

Fig. 6 Remember you're treating a person, not just an injury.

1. 'Have you had any operations in the past?'

2. 'Have you ever had any serious illnesses?' (In relation to this question, I ask specifically if the person is diabetic or epileptic.)

3. 'Are you allergic to anything?' (In particular, I ask for allergy to penicillin, and for hay fever or asthma.)

4. In the case of a woman, I ask for previous obstetrical and gynaecological history—i.e. how many babies has she had, any

miscarriages and any gynaecological operations. The First Aider will rarely find it necessary to go so deeply into a woman's previous history. However, it is possible that the First Aider may be faced with the task of delivering a baby, and when faced with the Emergency Childbirth Procedure, it is far more comforting to know that a woman has had three normal deliveries previously, than to know that she has had three previous Caesarean sections!

You may wonder why I ask the above questions in the above order. Well, there are many people who do not differentiate between illnesses and operations. After all, appendicitis is an illness, even though an operation may be necessary to cure it. However, an operation is a landmark in any person's medical history, because it takes place at a definite time. An illness may last for a variable time, from a few days up to a few months. Therefore by asking for operations first, we establish the landmarks, and at the same time, we isolate the previous surgical history (appendicectomy, etc.) from the previous medical history (pleurisy, duodenal ulcers, allergies, etc.) In any case, as I said before, I have found that this is the least time-consuming method of obtaining the previous history.

The information obtained from the history should be recorded as concisely as possible, because it can be of great value to the medical and nursing staff when the patient reaches hospital. In no case is this more true than in the case of a head injury history. Every scrap of information should be recorded, because the history may be the factor which determines whether or not the neurosurgeon has to operate.

5

The examination

The basic method of examining a patient is a time-honoured sequence which, as any doctor can tell you, is Inspection, Palpation, Percussion and Auscultation, in that order. In other words, we use our eyes for looking (Inspection), our hands for feeling (Palpation), we drum on the patient's chest or abdomen and listen to the note produced (Percussion) and we listen to breath sounds and bowel sounds (Auscultation). It is a common myth that the doctor's stethoscope is a magical instrument. In fact, it is possible to hear breath sounds more clearly by putting the ear directly onto the chest (this is known as Direct Auscultation), than by using a stethoscope (Indirect Auscultation). Actually, the use of the stethoscope is rather more polite than direct auscultation (especially when the patient is a young lady!), and it saves the doctor from having to perform acrobatics in order to listen to a chest. Basically, therefore, when examining a patient, we are using the natural senses with which we have been endowed, i.e. sight, touch and hearing. Sometimes we even use our sense of smell. For instance, we can detect the sweet-smelling breath of a diabetic.

Once we have taken the history and examined the patient, we use the information so obtained, and we then arrive at a diagnosis. It is often stated that experience is a great teacher, and the more experience we gain, the more quickly we are able to arrive at a diagnosis. Let us proceed with the examination.

The general condition of the patient

It is one thing to diagnose individual injuries, but it must always be remembered that the injury is attached to a person, and not the other way around. In other words, you are treating a *person* all the time, no matter what the injury, or injuries, may be. The main reason for splinting a fractured limb is to make transportation more comfortable for the person to whom the limb belongs. With this

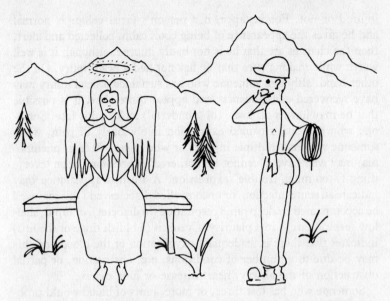

Fig. 7 Look for any 'give-away' altitudes.

in mind, we should always be aware of the general condition of the patient, because this will often be the determining factor in establishing priority of evacuation when dealing with mass casualties. It has been stated in many First Aid Manuals that the person who makes the most noise is the one who probably has the least injuries. This is often true, because he is still capable of devoting energy to a noisy display of anxiety. The person who is quiet, listless and often pale, is the one most likely to be seriously injured, because his energy is all being concentrated into trying to keep himself alive. He has no energy to spare for making a noise.

The five main factors which give us a good idea of the general condition of the patient are:
1. facial appearance
2. pulse
3. respiration
4. temperature
5. blood pressure.

I will deal with them in that order.

1. Facial appearance

An experienced person can often tell at a glance if a person is badly injured or not. For instance, if a person's facial colour is normal and he gives the appearance of being cool, calm, collected and alert, then the chances are that he is not badly injured, although it is well worth while making sure that he has not had a head injury. On the other hand, although someone who has sustained a head injury may have recovered consciousness and appear quite alert, it is possible that he may have a far-away (or 'yonderly') look on his face. Someone who exhibits a pained expression is obviously in pain, while someone who has multiple injuries or who is very ill (e.g. pneumonia) may well have a 'cannot-be-bothered' expression, or an 'everything-is-too-much-trouble' expression. A flushed appearance may indicate an acute infection, or uncontrolled diabetes, and this may well be accompanied by deep rapid respiration (in diabetes), or rapid, shallow respiration, as in a pleurisy. Cyanosis (a bluish tinge of the lips) indicates that there is inadequate oxygenation of the blood and this may be due to a number of conditions, e.g. obstruction, or partial obstruction of the airway, heart disease or lung disease.

Someone who has lost three, or more, pints of blood would probably have a worried, anxious look on his face and would probably have a pale, cold and clammy skin. If the blood loss were greater than three pints, he would develop dark rings under his eyes, become restless and exhibit rapid, shallow breathing, together with the signs of shock (see below). These signs having appeared, he would be in big trouble. If he were to go on to develop *Air Hunger* (i.e. deep, signing respiration caused by gross loss of red blood cells), then he would be in very serious trouble, because he would surely die, if he were not transfused with blood very soon.

Shock is a clinical condition characterised by pallor, a cold, clammy skin and a rapid, thready pulse, and these three signs are associated with a lowering of blood pressure. The causes of shock can be divided into three groups *viz*:

1. Cardiogenic shock—i.e. anything which affects the function of the heart. Examples of this type of shock are coronary thrombosis, pneumothroax, stove-in-chest and electric shock.

2. Neurogenic shock—i.e. anything which affects nervous control over the heart and vascular system, especially pain. For example, the 'Acute Abdomen' (perforated duodenal ulcer, appendicitis, strangulated hernia, etc.) causes pain, which in turn causes shock.

3. Vascular shock. This is caused by heavy fluid loss, such as blood loss from fractures, internal bleeding, or external loss from a severed artery. Burns may result in heavy plasma loss, and some-

times cause gross destruction of red cells. Intestinal infections may cause profuse vomiting or diarrhoea, resulting in a heavy loss of ECF, and heat stroke causes loss of ECF together with gross salt depletion. Vascular shock can be induced by any of these causes.

Pallor can also be the result of the adrenaline response to injury (this was mentioned in Part I). This form of pallor is usually associated with a *temporarily* raised blood pressure, and it occurs especially in young men within the first one to three hours after a serious injury. *Beware the pallor associated with a raised blood pressure after injury!* If the fracture is one from which three or more pints of blood can be lost, then eventually the blood pressure must come down to normal, and thereafter it will fall to below normal. Sometimes, the fall in blood pressure can be calamitously rapid, and therefore the injured person must have an intravenous drip set up as soon as possible (i.e. a sterile tube and needle put into a vein, to allow fluid to pass into his circulation). The reason for this is that, if his blood pressure does collapse suddenly, fluids can be pumped rapidly into his circulation to combat the fall in blood pressure and to restore the circulatory volume.

Well, that more or less takes care of facial appearance, except for the comment that some bright spark somewhere must make, 'You cannot detect pallor in a dark-skinned person!' Well, hard luck, Mr Bright Spark, your statement is incorrect. A certain amount of pallor *can* be detected in the face of a coloured person, who is ill or injured, and this is true for the vast majority of coloured people. The exception to the rule is the coloured person whose skin looks *very* black indeed, but even then, pallor can be detected. Look at the fingernails. Look at the insides of the lips and mouth, and at the inner sides of the lower eyelids. These places are a nice, healthy pink colour in a healthy person, regardless of his race. After heavy blood loss these places become pale, whether the person is coloured or not; the skin still feels cold and clammy and there is also a rapid, thready pulse.

2. The pulse

The pulse is really the impulse of a column of blood passing through an artery following the expulsion of blood from the heart during its contraction. The pulse most commonly felt for is the radial pulse. To feel your own radial pulse hold your right palm upwards. Now place the palm of your left hand against the back of your right lower forearm, just above the wrist, and then let your left fingers curl round onto the front of the lower end of your right radius (the forearm bone on the same side as the thumb). By exerting gentle pressure with your left fingers, you should be able to feel your right radial pulse with your left index, middle and ring fingers. If you now press down hard on the artery with your left ring finger, you will stop the blood flowing any further along the artery, and you will no longer feel the pulse with your left index and middle fingers. You will still feel it with your ring finger as the heart tries to pump blood past the obstruction. In other words, you have been able to compress the artery because it is soft and elastic (i.e. healthy). In old people, this is often not possible to do, because the arteries become dilated and hardened during the ageing process. The radial pulse is the one most commonly felt for, but there are other places where arterial pulses can be felt—the Femoral pulse in the groin, the Carotid pulse in the neck and the Superficial Temporal pulse just in front of the ear. Anaesthetists find the superficial temporal pulse very convenient to use because they usually sit at the head-end of the operating table.

We feel at the pulse in order to determine its *Rate, Rhythm* and *Volume. The pulse rate* is the number of beats per minute, which

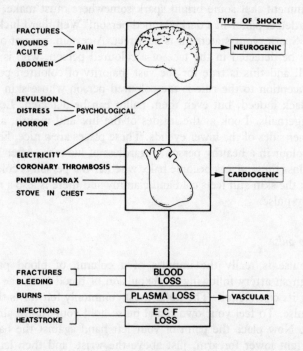

Fig. 8

can be determined with the aid of a watch with a seconds finger. The normal rate varies considerably. The resting pulse rate may be anywhere between fifty and ninety beats per minute. *The pulse rhythm* is normally regular, even after injury, although the pulse may become very rapid and extremely feeble in a person who reaches the stage of circulatory collapse. Irregularities can occur in heart disease, which does not usually concern the First Aider. What we mean by *the pulse volume* is the strength of the pulse. The normal volume of the radial pulse can be learned by feeling your own (as described above). You will also note that the femoral pulse has a greater volume than the radial pulse. This is because it is a bigger artery. For the same reason, the carotid pulse volume is greater than that of the radial artery, whilst the smaller, superficial temporal artery has a smaller pulse volume than any of the other three arteries mentioned.

Exercise (physical work, running, jumping, etc.) causes a normal increase in pulse volume and rate, because the heart has to pump out more blood per beat and at more beats per minute, in order to try to keep up with the body's increased energy consumption.

Abnormal increase in pulse volume occurs:

a. in the later stages of brain compression, after head injury.
b. in diabetic (ketotic) coma.
c. during the adrenaline response to injury.
d. in *acute* infections.

Please note, at this stage, that 'acute' means 'of rapid onset', and that 'chronic' means 'prolonged'. For example, tuberculosis is

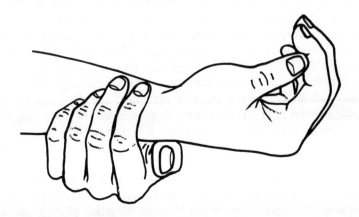

Fig. 9 Taking the pulse.

usually a chronic (prolonged) illness, whereas pneumonia is usually an acute illness (of rapid onset).

Abnormal reduction of pulse volume occurs:

a. typically after blood loss, when the pulse rate is increased, giving a typical *rapid, thready pulse*, together with a cold, clammy skin.

b. in hypoglycaemic (or insulin) coma, where the pulse is slow and weak, *after* unconsciousness has supervened.

c. in the initial stages of unconsciousness, the pulse may be rather slow and weak.

d. in a simple faint (otherwise known as vaso-vagal syncope), when at first, the pulse actually disappears for a few seconds and then begins to return. Initially, it is slow and very weak, but gradually the rate and volume of the pulse both increase until they become normal again, and the patient recovers consciousness.

The pulse *rate* and *volume* are the main concerns of the First Aider. The idenfitication of irregularities of rhythm is too complicated for First Aiders. The pulse rate is easily counted, but the recognition of the normal pulse volume (and, hence, of the abnormal pulse volume) demands PRACTICE, PRACTICE, PRACTICE. So practise, by feeling at other people's pulses, as well as your own.

3. Respiration

When considering respiration, we want to know its *rate* and *depth*. The normal, resting respiration is fairly shallow, and its rate is about 16–20 per minute. The rate and depth of respiration are both increased during exertion of any kind, of course, and this is normal. However, deep and fairly rapid respiration occurs, together with a rapid, bounding pulse (increased pulse volume) in diabetic coma, because the person in diabetic (ketotic) coma is trying desperately to breath out the poisonous ketones, which have built up inside him, and which are the cause of his coma. On the other hand, someone who is in a coma caused by an overdose of insulin (hypoglycaemic coma) will display rather slow and shallow breathing, together with a slow, feeble pulse. Air hunger has already been mentioned (see 'Facial Appearance'). It is very deep, sighing respiration and it occurs because of gross loss of red blood cells (i.e. tremendous blood loss). Because there are few cells left in his circulation, the injured person has to make the fullest possible use of his lungs in order to try to satisfy his need for oxygen. Therefore, he inhales and exhales fully, all the time. Obviously, such a person will be very pale, because the tremendous blood loss has thrown him suddenly into a severely anaemic state, and he will die soon unless he is transfused with *blood*, (at this stage, blood substitutes and plasma are inadequate, because they cannot compensate for the loss of the red cells).

There are two other kinds of respiration which should be mentioned:

a. Stertorous respiration. This is a rapid, shallow and noisy respiration. It is seen in chest injuries and, sometimes in abdominal injuries.

b. Cheyne-Stokes respiration. This is 'Crescendo breathing', in which the breathing gradually builds up from a slow and shallow stage to a rapid and deep stage. Then it gradually returns to a slow and shallow stage, after which period of *apnoea* (i.e. 'no breathing') follows. The pattern repeats itself, each crescendo being separated from the next by a period of apnoea.

When this Cheyne-Stokes form of respiration occurs, it is a sign that the person is near to death and beyond recovery—it is a *terminal sign*.

I have never known anyone survive once Cheyne-Stokes respiration has begun. It occurs commonly as a terminal sign in cases of head injury, although it could occur as a terminal sign in a case of diabetic (ketotic) coma.

Cheyne-Stokes respiration should not be confused with a type of respiration, which can occur in climbers at altitudes in excess of ten thousand feet above mean sea level. The climber may be breathing slowly and shallowly. Then suddenly, an outburst of deep, rapid respiration occurs, which tails off into slow, shallow respiration

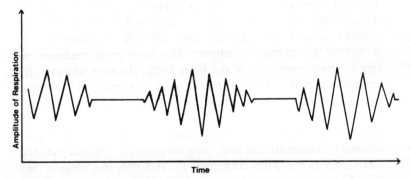

Fig. 10 Cheyne-Stokes respiration.

again within a few seconds. This type of high-altitude respiration should not be confused with Cheyne-Stokes respiration, because there is no gradual build-up of respiration to the deep, rapid stage. High-altitude respiration is the price, which Man pays for trying to exist at an altitude for which he is not designed.

4. Temperature

The temperature of the human body can be measured by using an oral thermometer, which can be placed into the mouth, or into the armpit. The most accurate reading is made by using a rectal thermometer. Special electronic rectal thermometers are now available, and they give a very accurate reading within seconds, where the usual mercury clinical thermometers take two or three minutes to give an accurate reading.

The normal *maximum* human body temperature is 37°C (98.6°F), but many normal, healthy people have temperatures of 36.1°C (97°F). The temperature of the body may be raised *slightly* after exertion, but any gross elevation of temperature occurs because of infection, heat stroke, or in the later stages of brain compression after injury.

Lowering of the body temperature (*hypothermia*) occurs in fell-walkers and mountaineers, as a result of exposure of the body to very cold conditions. Hypothermia can occur rapidly in people, who fall into extremely cold water, and it can occur in young babies and elderly people, for different reasons (see causes of unconsciousness, p. 87). Hypothermia means that a reduction of temperature has occurred in the *body core*.

At this point, I should explain that the modern concept of body temperature is that there is a *surface temperature* (i.e. skin temperature) and a *core temperature* (i.e. the temperature of the inner parts of the body). Now, on a cold day, the blood vessels in the skin constrict, in order to reduce heat loss, and so the skin temperature, or surface temperature is reduced. This is no great detriment, as long as the temperature of the inner body, the core temperature, remains at a healthy level. However, once a person's core temperature begins to fall, that person has begun to suffer from hypothermia. Special rectal thermometers, which give readings to well below those obtainable with the ordinary clinical thermometers, are necessary to measure the body core temperature. Ordinary clinical thermometers are quite inadequate for this purpose, because they record temperatures down to only 35°C (95°F).

5. *Blood pressure*

I have made mention already of blood pressure in Part I, and of the fact that exercise causes an increase in the systolic blood pressure, but little, if any, increase in the diastolic blood pressure. In fact, it may cause a *decrease* in the diastolic blood pressure. It can be seen, therefore, that exercise must increase the pulse pressure. The pulse pressure is also increased by the adrenaline response. A fall in blood pressure is usually the result of heavy blood loss, when it is associated with a rapid, thready pulse; but it also occurs in the final stages of brain compression (just before death) and in insulin coma. In each of these cases, the pulse will become progressively slower and weaker.

6

Measurement of blood pressure

The instrument which measures blood pressure is a sphygmomanometer, or 'sphyg' for short. There are two kinds of 'sphyg':

a. *The mercury sphyg*. This shows the blood pressure by means
of a column of mercury, in the same way as mercury barometer
shows atmospheric pressure.

b. *The anaeroid sphyg*. This functions basically like an anaeroid
barometer. Anaeroid means 'without air'. The anaeroid sphyg is
much lighter and more compact than the mercury sphyg, but it
should be checked regularly against a mercury sphyg to be sure
that it still reads accurately. If its accuracy decreases, it can be re-
calibrated.

I shall now describe how to use a sphygmomanometer. First of
all, there is a rather long piece of cloth which is to be wrapped
around the right arm half way between the shoulder and the elbow.
In one end of this cloth there is an inflatable cuff, and from this
cuff either one or two rubber tubes emerge through the cloth (one
or two tubes depending on who manufactured the sphyg and
when). The tube, or tubes, will eventually be connected to the
sphyg itself. The sphyg has a dial and below the dial there is a nut
which, when tightened up, will prevent air from escaping. When
loosened it allows air to escape. Below the nut there is a rubber bulb
which, when squeezed repeatedly, pumps air into the sphyg system.

Method (The internationally accepted method)

1. Bare the *RIGHT* arm of the patient, and make sure there is
no constricting object (e.g. a tightly rolled-up sleeve) which could
cause a false blood pressure reading. (N.B. Some sphygmomanometer manufacturers insist on describing the use of their sphygs on
the left arm, but the correct method is to use the right arm, unless
it has been injured or amputated).

2. Squeeze all air out of the inflatable cuff.

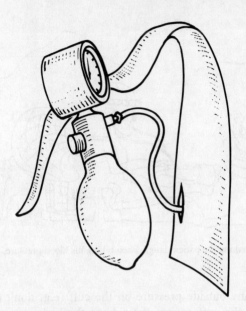

Fig. 11 Anaeroid sphygmomanometer and cuff.

3. Place the inflatable cuff on the inner side of the arm (over the brachial artery) half way between shoulder and elbow. Wrap the rest of the cloth round and round the arm so that it keeps the cuff firmly, but not tightly, in place against the brachial artery. Finally tuck in the end of the cloth to prevent it slipping. The cloth should *always* be wound round from the inner side of the arm, across the front; then the outer side, then the back and onto the inner side of the arm again. It should *never* be wound round the other way. Whilst applying the cuff, the patient's arm should be held straight out. He should not be allowed to bend the elbow as this may loosen the cuff. When the cuff has been applied, it should be a snug fit, and it should not be wrinkled up. The above description is that of the correct and internationally accepted way to apply a sphyg cuff. The *only* exception to the rule occurs when someone has either injured or lost the right arm, in which case the left arm has to be used, but the cuff is still wound round from the inner to the front, then to the outer side, then to the back of the arm.

4. Connect the tube to the connector on the sphyg.

5. Keep the patient's arm outstretched and tell him to relax his fingers, to breath normally and not to talk, laugh or cough, or hold his breath. (These actions can affect the blood pressure reading.)

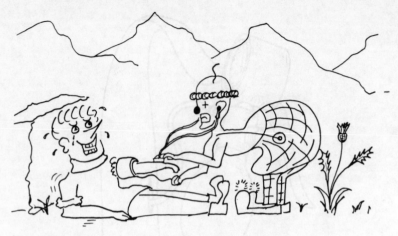

Fig. 12 Avoid making the patient laugh when taking his blood pressure.

6. Avoid any outside pressure on the cuff (e.g. don't allow the arm to press the cuff against the side of the body, or against the bed or your knee).

7. Place a stethoscope in your ears, in readiness. (A stethoscope from a child's nursing outfit is much lighter to carry around than a doctor's stethoscope and it is every bit as functional for the First Aider's requirements!)

8. Place the index and middle fingers of your *left* hand flatly across the inner side of the front of the patient's *right* elbow (this is where his brachial artery crosses his elbow).

9. Pump the sphyg bulb repeatedly and rapidly until the needle points to about 100 mm. You should now be able to feel his brachial artery pulsing away under your left index and middle fingers. *Keep your fingers there!* Do not lose that spot! Now, carry on pumping until the brachial pulse can no longer be felt. The pressure in the cuff is now greater than the patient's systolic blood pressure (the upper blood pressure reading) because it is preventing arterial blood from getting through to the forearm.

10. Now allow air to escape SLOWLY, by releasing the nut very slightly, and keep a sharp eye on the pointer. Note the reading on the sphyg when you feel the pulse return. This is the systolic blood pressure and this is the only way to find it—i.e. by feeling with your left index and middle fingers. You must NEVER listen for the systolic blood pressure before feeling for it. If you do listen, you *may* get away with it a few times, but eventually you will hear

sounds which will lead you to record a falsely high, or falsely low systolic blood pressure.

11. Having found the systolic blood pressure (by *feeling* for it) apply the chest piece of the stethoscope to the place where you felt the brachial pulse, and you will hear a 'Thump, thump, thump' as the blood passes through the artery. Keep the stethoscope there, and slowly release more air. The reading will fall, of course. When you hear a slight change in the force of the 'thump', note the reading. This is the diastolic pressure, and at about 5 mm below this reading, the thumps' should disappear altogether.

A word of caution here. You should watch the pointer on the dial and keep on listening until the pointer reads zero. The reason for this is that in some people (notably middle-aged men with somewhat raised blood pressures) the 'thump' sound appears at the systolic pressure, persists as the pressure reduces, then suddenly disappears, only to reappear later quite strongly, and then disappears later, just after the diastolic pressure has been reached, as described above.

The description of the steps to be taken may make the whole process seem to be a long one, but in fact, with practice, you will find that you can take a blood pressure in two minutes flat, or even less. Just one other thing I should mention and that is, that the blood pressure as recorded by one person may differ slightly from the blood pressure as recorded by another person. The reason for this is that we all have slightly different hearing abilities. For this reason, it is generally agreed that we record both systolic and diastolic pressures *TO THE NEAREST 5 mm* and, therefore, your reading should not differ by more than 5 mm from anybody else's reading. You can practise taking blood pressure on each other. It is possible to assess one's own blood pressure, but it is much easier to assess that of someone else.

Now that we have considered the foregoing indicators of the patient's general condition, we may proceed to the search for injuries.

7

The search for injuries

The examination has begun already by assessing the temperature, pulse, respiration, blood pressure and facial appearance. Apart from facial appearance, simple observation can reveal some 'give-away' attitudes. For example, in the case of a *fractured clavicle*, the patient typically inclines his head towards the injured side and hugs the shoulder of the injured side with the hand of the uninjured side.

In the case of a *dislocated shoulder*, the normal, rounded appearance of the Deltoid muscle (the muscle covering the upper, outer third of the humerus) can no longer be seen, and instead the Deltoid muscle is flattened out by comparison with the normal side. The injured side is supported below the elbow by the hand of the normal side, whilst the elbow of the injured side is semi-flexed. When the elbow is dislocated, there is loss of the normal bony triangle (this will be mentioned again, when I deal with injuries to bones and joints). The *dislocated elbow* is held semi-flexed and the limb is supported, just above the wrist, by the hand of the normal side. A similar attitude is adopted when there is a *supracondylar fracture of the humerus*. In *Colles' fracture*, as every First Aider knows, there is a typical 'dinner fork' deformity. In young children, a condition called *pulled elbow* may occur, (*to be described in Injuries to Bones and Joints*) and in this condition the whole of the upper limb hangs limply, because it is too painful for the child to lift that limb.

The 'give-away' attitudes of the lower limbs are, of course, those of the hip injuries. In *fractured neck of femur* (*NOT* impacted fracture of the neck of the femur), there is typically a shortening of the injured limb with the foot everted (turned outwards). In *dislocation, or fracture-dislocation of the hip*, the injured hip is held in flexion, internal rotation and adduction (pulled towards the midline), and the knee is therefore, held in flexion, so that the foot can support the weight of the limb.

So far, we have used our powers of observation (Inspection), but now we get round to feeling (Palpation). The patient may say that his thigh hurts, and there may be an obvious deformity of the femur. He may say he has pain in his leg, and there may be an obvious deformity of the tibia and fibula. Nevertheless, it is still important to feel for injuries, for the following three reasons, which are very basic but very important:

1. *Pain* is a purely personal sensation, and it is a *symptom*. A symptom is something of which the patient complains. Pain should not be confused with *tenderness*, which is a *sign*—i.e. something elicited on examination. Tenderness means that when we exert pressure over an injured area we cause pain. It is common to have a complaint of pain at a certain site and to be able to elicit tenderness at that site. However, it can happen that tenderness may be elicited at a site where the patient did not complain of pain.

2. Furthermore, if a patient has two injuries, he may be so distracted by the pain from the first site of injury that he does not complain of pain at the second site of injury. In such a case, the second site of injury is said to be '*masked*' by the pain from the first site.

3. A person may be injured in one place, and yet the pain of that injury may be felt in another place. This is known as 'referred pain'. The prize example of referred pain occurs when a person with a fractured neck of femur complains of pain in the knee on the same side (fractured neck of right femur, pain in right knee), but not of pain in the hip.

This phenomenon of referred pain can be explained by Hilton's Law. Hilton was an anatomist. He found that when a muscle acts upon a joint to alter the position of that joint, then both the muscle and the joint receive nerve fibres from the same nerve. The muscle receives motor nerve fibres to make it contract, and the joint receives sensory nerve fibres, which carry sensory impulses to the brain. These sensory impulses inform the brain of the joint's position, (whether the joint is flexed or extended). Now, the Quadriceps muscle on the front of the thigh helps to flex the hip and also to extend the knee, whilst the Hamstring muscles at the back of the thigh, help to extend the hip and to flex the knee. So, we have two groups of muscles, each acting on the same two joints. Therefore, using Hilton's Law, we can see how easy it is for the brain to confuse the two joints after injury. In fact, the brain is interpreting the pain as coming from the knee, when really the injury is in the region of the hip joint.

For the three reasons just stated, it is clear that every patient MUST be examined from head to toe, so that sites of *tenderness* will not be missed. Also, it is important not to miss fractures, which are painless temporarily, because of the Adrenaline Response (see p. 10). These fractures are revealed by finding deformity, abnormal mobility and, particularly, bony crepitus. With practice, you should be able to go over a patient from head to toe in two minutes.

Method

ALWAYS EXAMINE FROM THE PATIENT'S RIGHT SIDE, unless you are left-handed in which case it is permissible to place yourself to the left of the patient.

A certain amount of pressure must be applied with *flat* fingers to all parts of the head, and the limbs must be squeezed firmly all down their length in order to find tenderness. To give yourself a good idea of the correct amount of pressure to be exerted, place your fingers flat on the top of your head and press downwards until you can feel a definite pressure build up in the back of your neck. That is the correct amount of pressure to use when pressing or squeezing. It will elicit tenderness without causing damage. The exception to this rule occurs when a person is unconscious and *MAY* have a depressed fracture of the skull. In the unconscious patient, the scalp and skull-vault must be palpated *VERY GENTLY*, in order to find swellings or depressions only. The unconscious patient cannot tell you that you are causing pain, and there is no sense in adding to any depression already present in the skull-vault.

For the purpose of the following exercise, I will assume that the patient is conscious. Initially, as you practise on each other, you will find it beneficial to assume that consciousness exists. Most injured people are conscious when found, anyway.

1. Head and neck

Face the patient, and first, feel gently over the skull vault for lumps or depressions and for lacerations of the scalp. All of these can be missed if we simply look. They must be felt for. Even blood is not easy to see in the hair, especially if the hair is dark. Blood is sticky and will be transferred to your fingers and be seen.

Next, press firmly (as described previously) over *all* the skull vault, including the forehead, temples, mastoid bones (behind the ears) and the occiput (the lower part of the back of the skull). Use both hands at the same time and look for bleeding or CSF from the ears whilst you are feeling. Clotted blood should be wiped away from the ear. This helps to distinguish between bleeding from inside the ear and blood which has trickled into the ear from a scalp wound. Then press down onto the nose (unless it is obviously deformed and bleeding). After this, press on each cheek bone simultaneously and continue pressing along the *zygomatic arch* (the bony arch or ridge which passes from the cheek bone to just in front of the ear). When you reach the front of the ear, move downwards, one fingerwidth only. One finger of your right hand should now be on the patient's left jaw-bone-joint, and one finger of your left hand should be on his right jaw-bone-joint. These joints are called the temporomandibular joints, or TM joints for brevity. (Thank Goodness for abbreviations!) Now, ask the patient to move his jaw up and down and then from side to side. In each case you should feel the normal, smooth movement occurring in the TM joints. Any rough movement, or 'crunching' feeling in these joints is abnormal. Now feel firmly down the jawbone right to the point of the chin, for deformity, swelling or loss of normal contour, tenderness and, possibly, crepitus (see *Injuries to Bones and Joints*). Remember to look inside the mouth for lacerations to tongue or cheeks, broken or loose teeth, and for blood trickling down the back of the throat which would indicate bleeding from behind the nose. If the person has had a head injury, it is worthwhile taking note of the pupils at this stage (see *Head injury*).

Lastly we examine the neck. Press firmly on the vertebrae of the cervical spine, working downwards from the base of the skull. *If no tenderness is found*, check the neck movements. Tell him to put his chin onto his chest (i.e. *full flexion*), then to put his head right back (i.e. *full extension*). Now, tell him to turn his head *fully* to the left and then *fully* to the right (i.e. *full lateral rotation* to left and right). Finally, tell him to make his left ear touch his left shoulder and then to make his right ear touch his right shoulder (i.e. *full lateral flexion* of the neck to left and right). Note any restriction of movement. If tenderness is found initially, do *not* check the movements. Splint the neck forthwith. That completes your examination of the head and neck.

2. Upper limbs

Press with the flat fingers over the collar bones and shoulder blades. Next, squeeze the limbs, with the same amount of pressure, all the way down from the shoulder to the fingers. Squeeze both upper limbs at the same time. Note any sites of tenderness, which will be re-examined later in more detail, (described in *Injuries to Bones and Joints*). If no tenderness is found, complete the examination of the upper limbs by ensuring that the joints all pass through a full range of movements. If tenderness is found in one upper limb, complete the examination of the *uninjured* limb only, at this stage.

Testing for joint movements in the upper limb

a. *Shoulder*. The basic movements at this joint are:
 (i) Flexion—i.e. raising the arm forwards, to point directly upwards.
 (ii) Extension—i.e. the exact opposite of flexion.
 (iii) Abduction—i.e. raising the arm sideways, away from the body.
 (iv) Adduction—i.e. the exact opposite of abduction.
 (v) Internal rotation—i.e. rotating the humerus, so that the front of the elbow comes to face inwards, towards the body.
 (vi) External rotation—i.e. the exact opposite of internal rotation. Tell the patient to place his hands behind his back, with his fingers pointing up his spine (this is full extension, full internal rotation and adduction combined). Then, tell him to place his hands behind his head and to push his elbows right back (this is full abduction and extenal rotation, combined). Finally, tell him to raise his *straight* arms above his head and place the palms of his hands together (this is full extension). If he can perform all of these movements, then he has a full range of movements in the shoulders.

 b. *Elbow*. The movements of this joint are flexion, extension, pronation and supination. If the patient can touch the tip of his left shoulder with his left fingers, then there is full flexion at the elbow. If he can stretch his arm out fully, with his palm upwards, and if there is no forward angulation of the elbow, then he has a full range of extension at the elbow. Now, place the elbow at a right angle and tuck the elbow firmly into the patient's side. If he can maintain that position and turn his palm down so that it is parallel to the ground, then he has full pronation. If he can maintain that position and turn his palm upwards, so that it is facing, and is parallel to the sky, then he has full supination. If he can perform all four movements fully, then we simply say that he has a full range of movements (or full 'ROM') at the elbow joint.

 c. *Wrist*. The movements of this joint are flexion, extension,

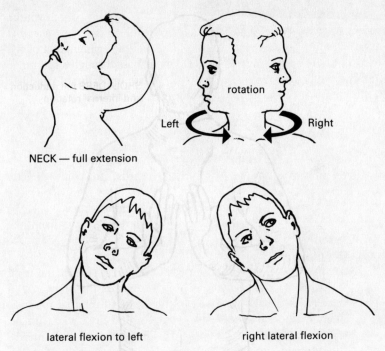

NECK — full extension

rotation

Left   Right

lateral flexion to left   right lateral flexion

Fig. 13 Neck movements.

adduction and abduction. If the patient can move the palm of his hand towards the front of his forearm so that an angle of 90° is formed, he has a full range of flexion. Likewise, if he can move the back of his hand towards the back of his forearm to form another angle of 90° he has a full range of extension. Now, tell him to place the hand straight in line with the forearm, and if he can then angle the hand towards the radial (thumb) side of the forearm to form an angle about 160° then he has full *ab*duction. If he can angle the hand towards the ulnar (little finger) side of the forearm to form an angle of about 140° then he has full *ad*duction. If he can do all these movements satisfactorily, then he has a full ROM at the wrist.

d. The hand.   This is very quickly tested. Ask the patient to make a fist and then to stretch out his thumb and fingers fully. If he can do this satisfactorily, there is not much need to worry about the hand. Any further examination of hand injuries should be carried out by a doctor who has special experience of hand injuries. That is important. The hand is far too intricate for a First Aider to be able to examine it in detail. *ALWAYS refer hand injuries for a medical opinion*, no matter how trivial the injury may seem to be.

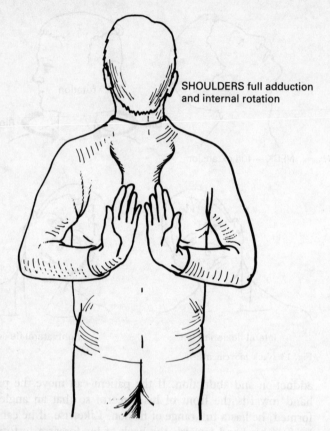

SHOULDERS full adduction
and internal rotation

Fig. 14 Shoulder movements.

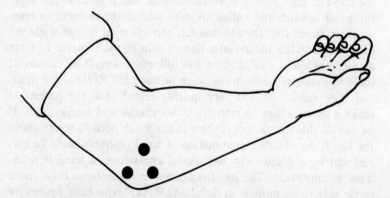

Fig. 15 The bony triangle of the elbow.

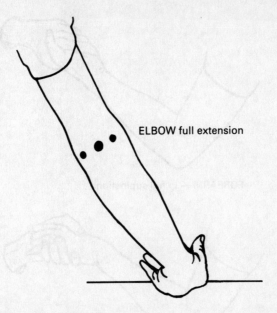

ELBOW full extension

Fig. 16 The bony triangle becomes a straight line (elbow fully extended).

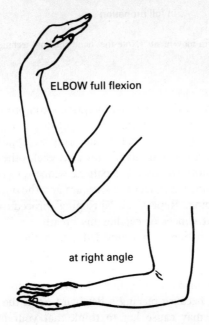

ELBOW full flexion

at right angle

Fig. 17 Elbow movements.

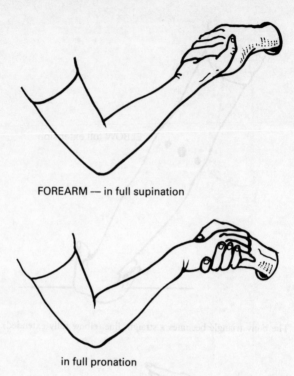

FOREARM — in full supination

in full pronation

Fig. 18 Forearm movements (Note the 'hand-shaking' technique).

3. The chest

The idea is to 'spring' the ribs by quickly compressing and releasing them. Place one hand on the left side of the rib cage and your other hand on the right side, below the armpits. Quickly compress the chest, by pressing your hands towards each other and release immediately. Note whether the patient winces or catches his breath. Now, place one hand over the sternum and the other over the dorsal (thoracic) spine. Repeat the 'springing' procedure and again note if the patient winces or catches his breath.

N.B. If the patient is a young lady, then the hand to be used on the sternum should be used as a 'clenched fist' and the soft part of the fist (the little finger side) should be the part to be placed on the sternum, because knuckles hurt. I advise you to use a clenched fist in this way, because placing a flat hand upon the front of a young lady's chest may cause her to think that your intentions are not entirely honourable!

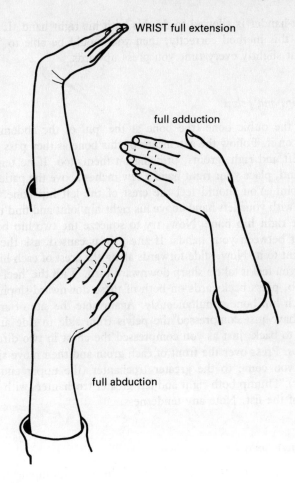

Fig. 19 Wrist movements.

4. Spine and sacrum

(a) Preferably, the patient should be asked to sit up for this (but see (b) below). With the patient sitting and leaning forwards, use the soft part of the fist to hump fairly heavily all down the dorsal (thoracic) spine, lumbar spine and over the Sacrum. Do not worry, you will not do any harm, and you will soon elicit any tenderness.

(b) If the patient cannot sit up then you will have to slide your left hand underneath the patient. Having done this, keep your fingers straight and press upwards with the tips of the fingers onto the spine. Repeat the process down the whole length of the spine.

A left-hander is allowed to do this with his right hand. If you are using this method correctly, then you should be able to 'lift' the patient slightly every time you press upwards.

5. Hips and pelvis

Find the pubic bone (the bone at the 'pit' of the abdomen) and press on it. Follow the extensions of this bone as they pass towards the left and right groins, pressing on them, too. If no tenderness is found, place your right hand a few inches above the patient's left hip joint. You should feel the crest of the left hip bone. Do the same with your left hand above his right hip joint and find the crest of the right hip bone. Now, try to squeeze the two hip bones together between your hands. If any pain is caused, ask the patient to point to it. Now, slide forwards along the crest of each hip bone, until you feel it take a sharp downward turn. With the 'heel' of each thumb, press backwards on both of these downward-sloping parts of each hip bone simultaneously. Again note the site of any pain. You have just compressed the pelvis from side to side and from front to back, just as you compressed the chest in two directions.

Hips. Press over the front of each groin and then move sideways until you come to the greater trochanter (the upper end of the femur). Thump both right and left greater trochanters with the soft part of the fist. Note any tenderness.

6. Lower limbs

You have begun the examination of these by thumping the hips. Now, quickly squeeze down the whole length of each lower limb (as you did with the arms) and note any sites of tenderness. If no tenderness is found, check the range of movements of the joints.

For the purposes of this exercise, let us assume that no tenderness has been found in the lower limbs. This means that we now have to check all the joints of the lower limbs for a full range of movements. Now, in order to test the ROM of the hip joint, the whole of the lower limb has to be moved. So, having squeezed your way down the lower limb to the toes, let us now work our way upwards again, through the joints of the lower limbs.

a. Toes. Simply push them all up together and then push them all down together. This is merely to see if there is any restriction of movement in one toe compared with the others.

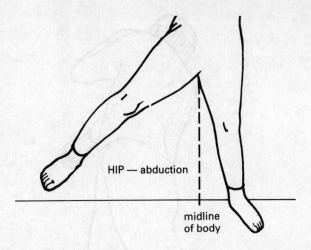

Fig. 20 Abduction of the hip.

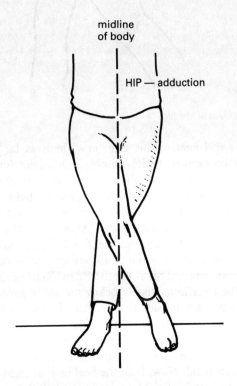

Fig. 21 Adduction of the hip.

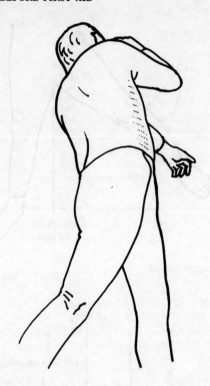

Fig. 22 Extension of the hip.

b. Mid-tarsal joint. This is a 'new' joint as far as most First Aiders are concerned. Quite simply, it is a joint formed amongst the bones of the tarsus and allows a small amount of rotation of the forefoot upon the hindfoot. To test this joint, hold the heel firmly in your left hand and then take hold of the forefoot, across the metatarsals, with your right hand. Now, twist the forefoot from side to side, trying to keep the heel fixed. You should find a range of movements which is about 5–10° either side of neutral.

c. Subtalar joint. This is another 'new' joint to most First Aiders. It is the joint immediately below the ankle joint, and it allows the heel to swing from side to side. It is the joint which enables us to walk on a surface which slopes sideways and therefore it is an important joint for slaters, tilers, property repairers, sailors and mountaineers. To test this joint, hold the leg firmly above the ankle with your left hand. Now, hold the heel in your right hand, making sure that the foot is at right angles to the leg. Swing the heel from side to side. Normally the heel moves, from the neutral position

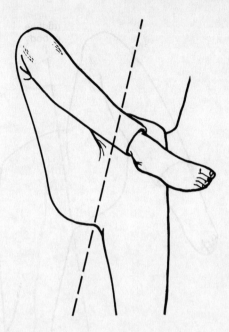

Fig. 23 External rotation of the hip (knee faces outwards)

about 10° towards the outer side of the leg and about 15–20° towards the inner side of the leg.

  d. Ankle joint. Everyone has heard of this joint! The test is easy, too. Push the foot upwards, towards the knee. This is called *dorsiflexion* of the ankle, and in full dorsiflexion, the foot should form an angle of about 80° with the leg. Now, push the foot downwards, away from the knee. This is called *plantarflexion*, and in full plantarflexion, the foot should form an angle of 180° with the leg.

  e. The knee. Full flexion of the knee forms an angle between the leg and the thigh of about 25–30° (in full flexion of the knee, you can more or less sit on your heel). In full extension, an angle of 180° (a straight line) is formed between the leg and the thigh.

  Approach the knee as follows:

 (i) Look and feel for swellings in or around the knee.
 (ii) Ask the patient to lift the heel off the ground and hold the knee straight. If he can do this, then:
(iii) Say, 'Keep your knee straight and do *not* let me bend it.'
(iv) Now, try to bend his knee. If the quadriceps muscle, at the front of the thigh is of normal strength, and if the patella is not damaged, you will not be able to bend his knee.

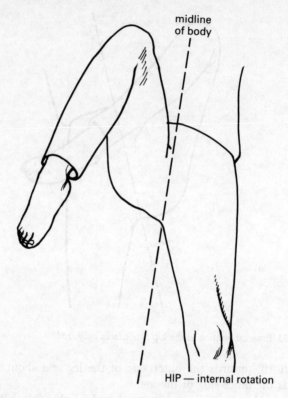

midline
of body

HIP — internal rotation

Fig. 24 Internal rotation of the hip (knee faces inwards).

(v) With the knee in the same fully extended position, try to bend it to either side. If the ligaments on either side are intact, the knee will not bend from side to side.

(vi) Finally, tell the patient to relax and see if the knee flexes (bends) fully.

If a First Aider can drill himself to examine a knee as well as that, then I shall be amply satisfied. It would be very unfair to ask a First Aider to examine a knee in any greater detail than I have described above. The examination for cartilage injuries is a difficult art which takes years of practice and experience to learn.

f. The hip. There are six movements which occur at this joint. They are:

(i) flexion—movement of the knee up towards the chest. Normally, the knee can touch the chest.

(ii) extension—the opposite direction. From the standing pos-

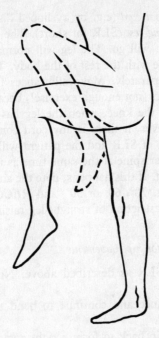

Fig. 25 Flexion of the hip.

ition, the thigh can normally swing backwards through about 30–40°.

(iii) abduction—movement of the lower limb away from the midline of the body. The normal maximum range of abduction is about 45°. Very supple people can achieve a much greater range than this (e.g. those who can do the 'splits').

(iv) adduction—movement of the lower limb towards and across the midline of the body. In other words, 'crossing one's legs'. The normal maximum range of adduction is about 35–40°.

(v) internal rotation. If you stand with your knees absolutely straight and then turn your feet inwards, you will find that your knee-caps are also facing inwards. Now, the amount of rotation which can occur at the knee and ankle is very slight indeed. Therefore, the movement must have occurred mainly at the hip. The normal maximum amount of internal rotation is 40°.

(vi) external rotation. This is turning the feet outwards. The normal maximum external rotation is 60°.

(vii) *Straight-leg raising*. Before I go on to describe the examination of the hip joint, I should explain that there is a *test for com-*

pression of the spinal cord (e.g. by a 'slipped disc'). This is called the *Straight-leg Raising test* (SLR for short). The straight leg is simply raised as far as it will go. The leg will normally go far enough to form a right angle with the rest of the body. The test is carried out with each leg separately. Make allowances for people with tight hamstring muscles (not enough exercise!) because they complain of tightness behind the knee, when the leg has been raised through about 80°. However, if there is any cord compression, then there will be limitation of SLR and the patient will complain of sudden pain in the lumbar spine at the same time as the limitation of SLR becomes apparent. If this happens, note the angle to which the limb was raisable, (e.g. 70°, 60° or 30°) and *RECORD IT*. (30° would represent gross restriction of straight-leg raising.)

The examination for hip movements

a. Carry out SLR as described above. Note any limitation or lumbar pain.

b. Bend the knee and continue to bend the hip till the knee touches the chest.

c. Bring the hip back to form a right angle with the body and, keeping the knee at a right angle also, swing the foot outwards, away from the midline. This is INTERNAL rotation of the hip joint. Note the angle which the leg (i.e. tibia) forms with the midline of the body.

d. Now, swing the foot in the opposite direction (across the midline). This is EXTERNAL rotation of the hip joint (the knee-cap points outwards). Note the angle which the leg forms with the midline of the body.

e. Put the first leg down straight and repeat (a) to (d) with the second leg.

f. Finally turn the patient onto the left side, place your left hand firmly on his pelvis, and pull each leg backwards in turn (the patient should be facing away from you now, if you are examining him from his right side, because you have turned him onto his left side). Note any restriction of extension. *N.B.* If you feel the patient's pelvis move, then you have reached the limit of extension of his hip.

7. The abdomen

This is the next in line for examination. I will not burden you with the details at this stage, because I have given you enough to be

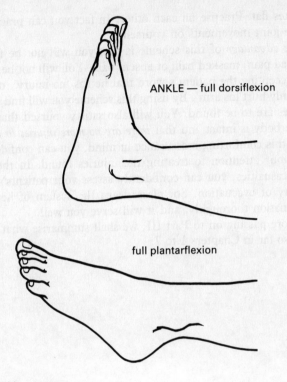

Fig. 26 Ankle movements.

practising already. For the time being, once you have completed the skeletal examination, just place a hand on the abdomen and say, 'Abdomen', so that you will train yourself not to forget! The examination of the abdomen will be dealt with in 'Abdominal Injuries'.

8. The chest (again!)

I know that we have been there already, but it may be necessary to take a closer look. More detailed examination of the chest is discussed in 'Chest Injuries'. For the time being, just put a hand on it and say 'Possibly chest'.

The foregoing description of head-to-toe examination may seem to be very long-winded indeed. If it does, then the reason is probably that most, or all, of the procedures mentioned are new to you. However, once you start to put the scheme into practice, you will find that each part of it takes far less time to do than to read, and eventually, your aim should be to cover the bones and joints in two minutes flat. Practise on each other. In fact you can practise most of the joint movements on yourself.

The advantage of this scheme is that you will not be fooled by referred pain, masked pain or absent pain. You will not be deceived into accepting the patient's word that he has 'no injury', or that he has 'only hurt his arm'. By using this scheme you will find whatever injuries are to be found. You will also satisfy yourself that the rest of the body is intact and that *there are no more injuries to be found*. With this comforting reassurance in mind, you can confidently devote your attention to treating the injuries found. In the case of mass casualties, you can confidently assess your patients' order of priority of evacuation. So, *please* learn the system of head-to-toe examination thoroughly, and it will serve you well.

Before passing on to Part III, we shall summarise what we have done so far in Chapters 1 to 7.

Summary of Parts I and II

In Part I, the normal function of the body was described. Much of Part I was necessarily factual. Facts are facts, and sometimes they have to be learned by sheer, hard slogging. There is no other way.

In Part II we developed the scheme of taking the history, assessing the general condition of the patient and examining the patient. I also mentioned a number of pitfalls to be avoided (e.g. NEVER simply accept the patient's word that he is 'alright'. ALWAYS satisfy yourself that he IS all right).

Now it may not always be essential to take the blood pressure, or to record the temperature, or even to count the rate of respiration. It is essential ALWAYS to feel and assess the pulse. This is good medicine.

So, let us recapitulate on the scheme we have developed.

The scheme (condensed)

1. Approach the patient with calm reassurance.
2. Start to take the history and, whilst the patient is answering you feel and assess the pulse and take a good look at his face (not so closely that you force him to ask what you are looking at!)
3. Look for any 'give-away' attitudes.
4. Go through the system of head-to-toe examination. Then examine sites of injury in greater detail.
5. Take the temperature, respiratory rate and blood pressure, where necessary.

Apart from developing the above scheme in your mind, I have given you (I hope) a great deal of food for thought. I have tried to give you the benefit of my experience in Part II, so it is up to you to take advantage of it.

In addition, I have described how to take a blood pressure and how to examine the whole of the skeletal system. I trust that you will practise these techniques regularly and as often as possible. In between your practice sessions, you can browse through Part III, *Specific subjects*.

Specific subjects

These specific subjects are those with which I dealt during a series of talks to the Rossendale Fell Rescue Team. At the end of the talks, I asked the team to take a test which I had prepared for them, and eighteen members of the team obliged. Now, the talks had lasted a total of ten to twelve hours. The object of the test was to find out just how well the team members had absorbed this concentrated bombardment of information. The test was mostly factual, but a few parts of it required ingenuity. The results were even better than expected. This made me think that if they could do so well in such a short time, then surely people elsewhere should be able to learn just as well, *provided* they could read the same information in their own good time, with each learning at his or her own individual rate of learning.

Depending upon your previous knowledge, you may be covering 'old ground' as you read through these subjects. Nevertheless, I hope that you will find them interesting.

A final topic which has been added onto this list of specific subjects is entitled, 'Mass casualties'. I hope that this will be of some benefit to search and rescue teams.

8

Causes of unconsciousness (and diagnosis of death)

There are quite a few possible causes of unconsciousness, and an apparently unconscious person may, in fact, be dead. Fortunately, there is an easy way to remember the common causes of unconsciousness. All you have to say to yourself is 'A,E,I,O,U and 3 Ds'.

Our shceme for remembering the causes of unconsciousness can now be written out as follows:

'A' — Apoplexy (i.e. stroke)

Asphyxia

Adder-bite (and the effects of other poisonous animals and plants, e.g. deadly nightshade)

Anaphylactic shock (anaphylaxis)

'E' — Epilepsy (and epileptiform convulsions, especially in children)

Embolism – i.e. massive pulmonary embolism (usually fatal)

Exposure – either to extreme cold or to extreme heat (e.g. heat stroke; burns).

Electric shock.

'I' — Injury—i.e. Head injury

Infarct—i.e. Myocardial infarct or Coronary thrombosis, or Heart attack

Infection—e.g. acute lobar pneumonia; malaria (especially the blackwater fever variety).

'O' — Overdose.

'U' — Uraemia, gross kidney malfunction.

'3 Ds' — Diabetes—hyperglycaemic or hypoglycaemic coma

Drunk—alcoholic intoxication

Dead

Shock

Simple faint.

I do not claim to be the originator of this scheme. It has been used for a long time. It is not one hundred per cent complete, and (as can be seen by comparison with the First Edition of this book) it can be shunted around and added to, to suit one's own purposes; but this list gives the common causes of unconsciousness, which the First Aider may well encounter and specific causes can usually be grouped under one of the above general headings. Let us now go over our scheme in rather more detail:

A

1. (i) APOPLEXY

Apoplexy or Stroke is caused by either a *cerebral haemorrhage* (i.e. bleeding into the brain tissue from a blood vessel) or a *cerebral thrombosis* (i.e. a blood clot blocking an artery in the brain tissue). In both of these conditions, the onset is usually quite sudden, and it usually leads to a complete paralysis of one side of the body—i.e. face, upper limb and lower limb. Because of weakness of the cheek on the affected side of the face, there is a typical 'blowing' sound as the patient exhales. The eyes often look towards the affected side of the brain (i.e. *away* from the affected side of the body) and the speech area may be affected (see '*Nervous System*' in Part I). The patient is typically elderly and may be conscious or unconscious.

Three other conditions which can be included under the heading of Apoplexy are Subarachnoid haemorrhage, Meningitis and Encephalitis. All three can result in unconsciousness

(ii) SUBARACHNOID HAEMORRHAGE

This occurs typically in young men in springtime. A *sudden* bleed takes place from the arterial system which surrounds the base of the brain; therefore the onset is sudden. A typical history would be, 'He was bending down to tie his shoe laces, when he suddenly fell to the floor unconscious'. The breathing is often deep and may be stertorous (noisy). The limbs are often rigid, but may be flaccid. The pupils are sometimes unequal and show a tendency to vary in size independently of each other. However the typical finding is *neck rigidity*. If you place your hand behind his head and try to bend his neck so that his chin touches his chest, you will not be able to do so. You may even lift him half way into a sitting position but you not be able to bend his neck. This is *true* neck rigidity. *It is a sign of irritation of the meninges* (the coverings of the brain and the spinal cord). In this case, it is caused by the bleeding which has occurred *outside* the brain tissue, but *inside* the meninges.

(iii) MENINGITIS AND ENCEPHALITIS

These occur typically in children, though any age-group may be affected. From the First Aider's point of view the two are indistinguishable. The onset takes place over a few days. The child complains of feeling unwell, may complain of a sore throat and becomes lethargic. A temperature develops and increases until the child looks flushed and feels very hot when you feel at his forehead, and he is very likely to be vomiting at this stage. Again, the typical finding is neck *ridigity* which, in this case, is caused by inflammation of the meninges by the infection. *N.B.* Do not mistake *meningism for neck ridigity*. Meningism occurs quite commonly in such conditions as influenza. The patient complains that his neck feels stiff, but his neck can be bent forward and his chin can be placed upon his chest though it may cause him a little discomfort.

When feeling at the forehead to see if it feels hot use the skin on the backs of the middle bones of your fingers. This skin has better temperature appreciation than the skin on any other part of the hand.

When meningitis is well advanced, the patient may arch his back spontaneously. This is called Opisthotonos and it may be so severe that the patient may be arched upwards, supported only by his head and heels.

2. ASPHYXIA

This is caused by anything which prevents the normal exchange of oxygen and carbon dioxide in the lungs. The causes can be divided into physical and chemical. The *physical causes* include such things as smothering, strangulation and inhaled foreign body—i.e. anything which physically prevents the air from passing into or out of the lungs. The *chemical causes* include poisoning by gases such as carbon monoxide and hydrogen cyanide (Prussic acid). These chemicals are able to combine very strongly with the haemoglobin in the red cells and having done so, they block the ability of haemoglobin to combine with either oxygen or carbon dioxide. The result of this is that the body suffers from lack of oxygen. *The treatment* of asphyxia is to remove any physical cause, give mouth-to-mouth resuscitation where necessary, and to remove the patient to hospital, especially when poisonous gas is suspected to have caused the asphyxia.

3. ADDER BITE (Common British Viper)

This topic introduces us very briefly to the immense subject of toxicology. This is the study of substances which are toxic (i.e. poisonous) to humans. *Venom* is the correct name for the poison produced by a snake, and although there are many kinds of poisonous snake, their venoms form only a small fraction of the many thousands of substances toxic to humans. Basically, there are three types of snake venom, namely:

a. Haemorrhagic venoms—these break up red blood cells and cause multiple small widespread haemorrhages.

b. Haemocoagulant venoms—these cause red blood cells to clot.

c. Neurotoxic venoms—these attack the nervous system, causing salivation, hallucinations, convulsions, respiratory paralysis and, ultimately, death.

Some venoms are mixtures of two of the above (e.g. neurotoxic and haemorrhagic).

All vipers produce venom in proportion to their body weights. For any given species of viper, the heavier the viper, the more venom it can hold in its venom sac, and therefore the more dangerous that viper is. Weight for weight, a newly-born baby viper is just as venomous as its parents. Likewise, the venom affects humans in a dose-to-weight ratio. Thus, in general, the larger the human, the less serious are the effects of a given dose of venom. Therefore, as a generalisation, children are more likely to suffer serious effects from snake bite than are adults. However, it must be pointed out that the venom of some vipers is so deadly that a few drops can kill a human adult in a few seconds, even if it is injected into soft tissues, because its absorption into the bloodstream from soft tissues is very rapid. Fortunately, the venom of the adder (C.B.V.) is absorbed very slowly from soft tissues, usually over a period of days rather than seconds. Other adders (e.g. the Puff Adder and the Death Adder) produce far more deadly venoms than the C.B.V.

The adder (Common British Viper or Viper berus) is the only naturally occurring poisonous snake in the British Isles. Typical of the vipers, it bears a V-shaped mark on its head and dark, zig-zag markings down its back. It grows to a length of about 30 cm (12 in) and rarely exceeds 45 cm (18 in). Like its closest relative, the Common European Viper which it resembles very closely, it produces a *haemorrhagic venom* whereas the American rattlesnakes (30 different species) all produce *neurotoxic* venoms. Despite its name, the Common European Viper is to be found in Asia and Japan as well as in Europe.

The adder tends to inhabit quiet forest glades and high, remote moorland, as far away as possible from humans. This seems to be a good recipe for the survival of both humans and adders. It probably accounts for the fact that an average of only one person per year in the U.K. sustains an Adder bite, with a resulting mortality rate of only 4 per cent. In the U.S.A., between 2 and 3000 people per year sustain rattlesnake bites, but the death rate is less than 1 per cent. In Brazil, the annual death rate alone from snake bite is 2000, and similar figures apply to Burma and Malaysia. Clearly, these countries have much more venomous snakes than the U.K. and the U.S.A., although the rattlesnakes are not the only poisonous snakes in the U.S.A.

In the U.K., therefore, we are relatively fortunate with respect to snake bite. Indeed, more people in the U.K. die per annum after bee-stings than after adder bites. Nevertheless, adder venom can be lethal, especially if injected directly into a vein. To stress the potential danger of adder venom, I will relate a true story. A game warden in Scotland lay down in a field one sunny afternoon for a nap. An adder came along and nestled up to him. He must have disturbed the adder because it bit him. The venom went directly into the axillary vein (the vein in the armpit, or axilla) and from there passed rapidly round the circulation. The game warden must have died quite rapidly, because he was found still lying in the field. Autopsy revealed numerous haemorrhages throughout the body, especially in the brain. This rare and very unfortunate case serves to emphasise the dangerous nature of the adder.

It has been postulated that the adder has two distinct types of bite, namely:

a. *A warning, or 'keep off the grass' bite.* This is a nasty nip, *without the* active injection of venom into the wound. It is used when the adder is startled by a human.

b. *A lethal, or 'business' bite.* This is a bite *with* the active injection of venom into the wound. It is used when the adder is annoyed, e.g. by a human who persists in trying to capture the adder.

This concept could apply also to the rattlesnakes of the U.S.A.

and could well account for the relatively low mortality rates in both the U.K. and the U.S.A. It is certainly an interesting concept.

Before going into the symptoms, signs and treatment of adder-bite, I must mention another interesting point about the adder. The adder is *not* a natural inhabitant of Ireland. Legend has it that when St Patrick arrived in the Emerald Isle, his first act was to drive all the serpents into the sea. Whatever the basis of this legend may be, the fact remains that there are no naturally occurring poisonous snakes in Ireland.

Symptoms and signs

Males seem more inclined to try to capture adders than females. This explains why males are twice as likely as females to suffer adder bite. It explains also the fact that a male tends to receive a bite to the hand or wrist, whereas a female is usually bitten on the ankle or leg. The sudden fright of having been bitten may cause *neurogenic shock and fainting*, from which the victim recovers in a few minutes. The usual complaint is of *quite severe pain* in the wound, where swelling occurs because of oedema (an excess of fluid in the soft tissues). A few hours later, *small haemorrhages may occur along the lymphatics* of the wounded limb, and *abdominal pains, nausea* and *vomiting* may occur. *Anaphylactic shock* (q.v.) may occur up to three days after the bite and, for this reason, *the adder-bite victim should be admitted to hospital for observation for a minimum of three days, even if he states that he feels perfectly well*. After a few days, the *wound sloughs* and the healing process may last for six weeks or more.

Prevention

This is obvious. *AVOID DELIBERATE CONTACT* with adders and any other poisonous animals and plants. If you are not a herpetologist who has been specially trained to handle reptiles, '*KEEP OFF THE GRASS*'!

Precaution

On arrival in a country which is known to have poisonous snakes, ask the local experts what to do in the case of snake-bite *BEFORE* it happens.

Treatment

(i) Lie the victim down and calm him down. Physical activity and anxiety both increase the circulatory rate, and this will increase the uptake of venom from the wound by the bloodstream. The object of lying him down and calming him down is to reduce uptake of venom to a minimum by keeping the circulatory rate to a minimum. If he feels more comfortable in the semi-recumbent ('propped up') position than lying flat, then this position should be adopted. It may be necessary to give Diazepam 10 mg by intramuscular injection in order to calm him. (Diazepam is produced under various trade names.)

(ii) The experts do *not* recommend the use of a tourniquet for adder bite. The reasons given for this are:
   a. The adder venom is absorbed relatively slowly from the soft tissues. Therefore a tourniquet will have little significant effect on the rate of absorption of venom.
   b. If the venom has been injected directly into a vein, it is too late to use a tourniquet.
   c. A tourniquet increases venous congestion and underoxygenation of the wound itself. This results in a larger area of wound sloughing and delayed healing of the wound.

(iii) Similarly, the experts do *not* recommend incision of the wound and sucking out the venom, because of
   a. increased wound damage by the incision and
   b. increased likelihood of absorption of venom via small blood vessels severed by the incision.

N.B. Having said all this, I must point out that the use of a tourniquet, incising and sucking the wound, and even the immediate amputation of the affected part (e.g. a finger) may well be life-saving measures after a bite from a tropical snake. The venom of the King Cobra, for instance, can be absorbed from soft tissues into the bloodstream so rapidly that it can kill within fifteen seconds.

(iv) The victim of adder bite should always be transported to hospital. *Never* allow him to walk. Walking increases the circulatory rate, which increases the rate of absorption of venom. In hospital, he should be kept under observation for at least three days because of the possibility of anaphylactic shock.

(v) Zagreb antivenom is effective against both Common European Viper and adder venoms. It can be given with safety to non-allergic people, but it can cause anaphylactic shock in people with a history of allergy (e.g. hay fever). If an allergic person is to be given Zagreb Antivenom, then adrenaline, an antihistamine and possibly hydrocortisone must be given first, in order to avoid anaphylactic shock. Therefore, some experts prefer to withhold Zagreb Antivenom from allergic people, unless it is absolutely essential to give it.

N.B. a. After snake bite, it is always helpful if the snake responsible for the bite can be killed and presented to the experts for identification so that the correct antivenom can be chosen. This is particularly important in the tropics, where there are many different antivenoms for the many different types of poisonous snake.

   b. *NEVER* handle the head of a dead poisonous snake. Even the head of a *decapitated* poisonous snake can deliver a lethal bite for up to twenty-four hours after decapitation. YOU HAVE BEEN WARNED!

4. ANAPHYLACTIC SHOCK (or 'systemic anaphylaxis')

This is an extremely severe hypersensitivity response to a foreign substance. Many substances are capable of causing it, e.g. penicillin, snake venoms (see 'Adder bite') and pollens. If we take penicillin as our example, we can divide people into four groups:

Group 1. Those who suffer no adverse effects whatsoever. This is the largest group.

Group 2. Those who suffer minor adverse effects (e.g. a sore tongue and/or antibiotic diarrhoea). This is the second largest group. The sore tongue and antibiotic diarrhoea are corrected quite easily by giving vitamin B compound tablets.

Group 3. Those who suffer an allergic reaction (i.e. a blotchy rash all over the skin and perhaps puffiness of the hands, feet and face). This is the third largest group. Antihistamines or even hydrocortisone may be needed to treat the allergic reaction. The allergy is acquired by repeated administration of penicillin over a period of time. Once this allergy has revealed itself, it is dangerous to give further doses of penicillin, because continued administration of penicillin, even intermittently, will eventually provoke anaphylactic shock.

Group 4. This is the minority group and, fortunately, a very small minority indeed. These people have an *inborn, extreme hypersensitivity* to penicillin. On receiving their *very first dose of Penicillin* they suffer anaphylactic shock. The enzyme, penicillinase, is now available for the treatment of penicillin-induced anaphylactic shock.

Penicillinase breaks down Penicillin into harmless chemicals.

Anaphylactic shock is characterised by the sudden onset of *bronchospasm* (constriction of the breathing tubes), *oedema of the larynx* (soft-tissue swelling of the voice-box), *breathlessness, cyanosis* (blueness of the lips and face because of under-oxygenation of the blood), *a very rapid weak pulse* and a *marked fall in blood pressure. Nausea, vomiting* and *diarrhoea* may occur also.

Multiple small haemorrhages may occur and the *vomitus may contain blood* if the anaphylactic shock is snake-venom induced, because some snake venoms are haemorrhagic (see *Adder bite*). If not treated promptly, anaphylactic shock is fatal.

Treatment consists of:

(i) *Treatment of hypoxia* (lack of oxygen). The bronchospasm reduces the amount of air which the patient can inspire; but, since inspired air normally contains about 21 per cent oxygen, the administration of pure oxygen increases the patient's reduced oxygen intake by nearly 400 per cent.

(ii) *Treatment of the anaphylactic reaction.* A combination of adrenaline, hydrocortisone and an antihistamine, given either by a doctor or under the supervision of a doctor, helps by reversing the reaction, raising the blood pressure, reducing the pulse rate, improving the pulse volume and eliminating the bronchospasm. The general condition of the patient is thus improved.

(iii) Neutralisation of the prime causative factor, *where possible.* If the causative factor is known, and if there is a specific antidote, then the antidote should be used – e.g. penicillinase if the causative factor is penicillin, or the appropriate antivenom for snake-venom-induced anaphylactic shock. Often, as with pollens, there is no specific antidote, in which case, the treatment consists of (i) and (ii), as above.

'E'

1. (i)   EPILEPSY

This is a condition characterised by intermittent convulsions. It is *not* familial. The commonest cause is brain damage at birth, though there are quite a number of possible causes, e.g. when epilepsy occurs for the first time during adult life, it is usually as the result of a severe head injury. *Very occasionally* it may be the first sign of a brain tumour. Please note that I said 'very occasionally'. So, do not go around diagnosing brain tumours right, left and centre!

The typical sequence of an epileptic attack begins with the Aura, followed by the Tonic phase, the Clonic phase and Flaccid phase, in that order. *The aura* is the warning phase, which often lasts only 15–30 seconds. During this phase, the patient knows he is going to have a fit, but he cannot warn anyone. Those who know the patient well may notice a certain vague appearance on his face and can prepare for the convulsion.

The tonic phase occurs suddenly. The patient falls to the ground and all his muscles tense up; he becomes completely rigid, not even breathing. He may become blue in the face (cyanosed), because this stage may last half to one minute. His face usually assumes a grimace.

The clonic phase occurs next. All the muscles of the body twitch violently, repeatedly and independently of each other. This may last up to two minutes, and it is during this phase that he froths at the mouth. He may pass urine and even faeces, because he has lost voluntary control of his bladder and bowels.

The flaccid phase takes over from the clonic phase. He relaxes, breathes more normally, though maybe heavily at first, and appears to be asleep. His colour returns to normal. This stage *may* last ten minutes or even more, though it may be over within a minute.

N.B.) (a) *Automatism* may occur sometimes after an epileptic fit. This is a state in which the patient appears to have returned to normal, but he performs automatic actions, e.g. going for a bus ride. This state may last for up to twenty-four hours. For obvious reasons, an epileptic must not be left alone for twenty-four hours after a fit. (b) *Status epilepticus* is a condition where one fit occurs and before the patient has fully recovered from it, another one begins and this is followed by another, etc. It is a series of fits strung together. If this occurs, you must get the patient to hospital or he will die.

(ii) EPILEPTIFORM CONVULSIONS

These commonly occur in children, but could occur in adults. A very high temperature causes spontaneous triggering-off of nervous impulses in the brain and the result is a convulsion, which may be followed by more convulsions. The most effective first-aid measure is to tepid-sponge the patient *all over*, to bring down the temperature. If the temperature is brought down and *kept down*, the convulsions will stop.

2. EMBOLISM

An embolus is a blood-clot, which commonly forms in a vein of a lower limb or in a vein in the pelvis. When the clot breaks free, it can travel along in the bloodstream towards the heart. A very small embolus will'pass through the right atrium and right ventricle and will lodge finally in a lung. A *massive* pulmonary embolus will lodge in the pulmonary artery. Thus, it will stop the flow of blood through the lungs and the victim suffers from lack of oxygen. Therefore, he collapses suddenly, becomes cyanosed and unconscious and will be very fortunate if he survives. So get him to hospital immediately!

3. EXPOSURE

This involves us in the results of exposure to extreme cold (the hypothermias and frostbite) and the results of exposure to extreme heat (heat syncope, water depletion, salt depletion and heat stroke), and the results of exposure to altitude (acute mountain sickness). First, we must consider the relevant physiology.

Relevant physiology

(i) Thermoregulation

This is the process by which the temperature of the body 'core' is maintained at a healthy level. The healthy *range* of body 'core' temperature is 36°C to 40°C (96.8°F to 104°F), depending upon the individual and the level of activity, because activity increases body 'core' temperature. Outside this healthy temperature range, functions of the body go very much astray. Body heat is produced as a by-product of metabolism, and this heat provides the body 'core' with its temperature; but, in order to maintain the correct body 'core' temperature, it is essential to be able to regulate the amount of heat lost, or conserved. This function is provided by the part of the brain known as the thermoregulatory centre. It responds mainly to the temperature of the blood, but also to stimuli from other parts of the body. It collects and collates information and then sets in motion a programme of heat conservation, or heat loss, depending on which is required at a particular time. It is part of the autonomic nervous system, and we have no voluntary control over it.

Heat loss can be achieved by one, or a combination, of the following means:

a. *Conduction.* This is the process by which heat passes directly from a warm object to a cold object where the two objects are in contact. For instance, if you leave your warm hand in contact with snow for a few minutes, your hand will become cold and some of the snow may melt because heat will pass directly from your hand to the snow. If you splash yourself with cold water on a hot day, you become cooler, but the water becomes warmer because it has absorbed heat from you.

b. *Radiation.* This is the process by which heat radiates from an object to the surrounding atmosphere. For example, you can feel the heat from a radiator without actually placing your hand upon it. Similarly, heat can radiate from the human body, especially after strenuous exercise, and this heat can be felt by another person standing nearby, without actual contact.

c. *Convection.* This is the process by which heat is removed from the surface of an object by a current of air (or any gas for that matter). A gentle breeze on a hot summer day can have a very pleasant cooling effect.

d. *Evaporation.* When a liquid evaporates from a surface, then that surface cools. This (like conduction, radiation and convection) is a principle of general physics. The body can use this principle by producing sweat. Sweat is a very dilute solution of salt. It is secreted actively onto the body surface by sweat glands. When the sweat evaporates, the body surface cools.

The thermoregulatory centre uses the latter three of these principles. By means of nervous impulses it can bring about dilatation of the blood vessels of the skin which increases the amount of warm blood passing through the body 'shell'. This results in increased heat loss from the body, by radiation and by convection. If still further heat loss is required, the thermoregulatory centre initiates sweating (via nervous impulses to the sweat glands), and evaporation of sweat provides extra heat loss. If even further heat loss is required, then the answer is cold water (e.g. a cold shower), which provides cooling by conduction of heat from the body to the water from the shower.

Heat conservation is achieved by the thermoregulatory centre, too. By stopping the sweating process, evaporative heat-loss is stopped. (However, it must be remembered that other liquids, such as rain and condensed mist, can evaporate from the body surface, providing *unwanted* heat loss.) The thermoregulatory centre can also cause a shut-down of the blood vessels in the skin, thereby minimising heat loss by radiation, convection and conduction. This reduction of heat loss (by radiation, convection and conduction) can be assisted greatly by wearing appropriate clothing and by insulating ourselves properly from any cold surface with which we may come into contact (e.g. lying down on frozen snow). Clothes add to the insulating effect of subcutaneous fat (i.e. the layer of fat under the skin). If, despite skin vessel shut-down and clothing, the body 'core' temperature drops just below 36°C (96.8°F), the thermo-regulatory centre initiates the process of *shivering*. This is a series of rapid, involuntary, muscular contractions, designed to consume *energy* rapidly, and thereby produce extra heat, which provides a quick boost to the body 'core' temperature. Provided that a person can still shiver, then that person is NOT in a hypothermic state.

(ii) Metabolism

In a nutshell, this means the production and use of energy. The *metabolic rate* is the *rate* of consumption of energy. It can be measured in terms of calories (i.e. kilocalories) consumed per hour. The metabolic rate of an individual varies according to activity, the lowest possible rate being known as the *basal metabolic rate* (or B.M.R.) which can be measured with the individual in a completely resting state. The maximum rate of consumption of energy is known as *the maximal metabolic rate* (or M.M.R.) and this, too, can be measured. The difference between the M.M.R. and the B.M.R. (in terms of calories) is the amount by which a person is capable of increasing his energy consumption above his B.M.R., and this is known as the *metabolic reserve* (or M.R.) Since a person is very rarely at complete rest, and since it is impossible to maintain the M.M.R. for more than a few minutes, the actual metabolic rate of a person, at most times, is somewhere between the B.M.R. and the M.M.R., and it varies, upwards or downwards, with changes in activity. Activity varies according to occupation. For example, a sedentary worker may consume only 1500 to 2000 calories per day, whereas a heavy manual worker may consume between 3000 and 5000 calories per day.

The different metabolic rates vary also according to age and sex. Women, in general, have lower metabolic rates than men. Babies, of course, consume less total energy than adults. Therefore, their *actual* metabolic rates are lower than those of adults; but when we consider the energy consumption of a baby *in relation to its weight*, then we find that its *weight-related B.M.R.* is greater than that of an adult. The reason for this is that a baby grows at a tremendous rate. On average, a baby doubles its birth weight in the first three months of life and trebles its birth weight in the first year of life Adults, on the other hand, have ceased to grow and need only to replace their daily energy consumption. *A baby's energy consumption is reflected in its food consumption, which again, on a weight-for-weight basis, is a relatively greater food consumption per day than that of the vast majority of adults.*

Since a very young baby's energy is mostly devoted to increasing the size of the baby, the baby has a high B.M.R., but a low M.R. The liver of the young baby is not as mature as an adult liver, and therefore it cannot store food products on a scale comparable with that of the adult liver. A young baby's heat conservation mechanism is poorly developed compared with that of an adult, and so the baby can become cold quite quickly. Therefore, frequent feeding and adequate clothing are necessary to provide energy and insulation, respectively, and thereby avoid hypothermia in babies.

As babies enter childhood and become increasingly mobile, the rate of growth declines, and, with it, the weight-related B.M.R., whereas the M.M.R. and M.R. increase. These changes progress up to early adult life, where the B.M.R., M.M.R. and M.R. tend to stabilise for a few years. At about twenty-eight years of age, we have reached our 'peak', the ageing process begins and the B.M.R. assumes a slow decline towards old age. The M.M.R., however, is still variable. If a person keeps fit, by training, the M.M.R. can be maintained, or even increased. This explains the fact that many marathon runners are at their best after the age of twenty-eight years. If a person does not train, the M.M.R. tends to decline. At first, this decline will be parallel to the fall in B.M.R., but if lack of training persists, the M.M.R. will decline more rapidly than the B.M.R. leading to a reduced M.R.

The relentless decline in B.M.R. continues past middle-age into old age, and there is a tendency for the M.M.R. to decline also, but the decline in M.M.R. can be minimised by physical activity, so that whereas one man in his sixties may be barely able to climb the stairs of his house, another man in his eighties may still be able to climb mountains. Eventually, however, even the fit eighty-year old will have to resign himself to the reduced, and still reducing, activity of extreme old age in which there is a very low B.M.R. together with a very low M.M.R. and, therefore, a very low M.R. When extreme old age is reached, it is difficult for the person to keep warm, even during a British summer, without considerable amounts of clothing. In winter, particularly, many such people sit close to a fire, heavily clothed, in order to keep warm, and some dare not even go out of the house during the winter months, so great is their fear of the cold.

(iii) Liver function

The liver is both the 'warehouse' and the detoxification centre of the body.

As the body's 'warehouse', it stores the food-products (carbo-hydrates, fats and amino acids) which have been obtained via the digestive system. When required, the liver can release these food-products into the bloodstream for transportation to other parts of the body where they are needed. Glucose is a particularly important carbohydrate because it is our main source of energy. Glucose is a soluble sugar. The liver stores it by converting it into glycogen which is an insoluble sugar. When the muscles increase their de-mand for glucose, the liver converts glycogen into glucose, which is then released into the bloodstream.

As the body's detoxification centre, the liver detoxifies (i.e. renders harmless) many substances which are harmful to the body—e.g. bacterial toxins. Some of the by-products of metabolism are harm-ful to the body, one very good example being ammonia which is obtained from the breakdown of amino acids. If ammonia were al-lowed to accumulate in the blood, it would have serious, and eventu-ally fatal, consequences. The brain is particularly susceptible to the effects of ammonia. The liver detoxifies ammonia by converting it to the harmless product, urea, which is then excreted by the kidneys.

If the temperature of the body 'core' (and with it the temperature of the liver) falls then all the functions of the liver are impaired—i.e. storage of food-products, release of food-products and detoxifi-cation of the harmful by-products of metabolism and other toxins.

(iv) Respiration

The vital part of this process is to obtain oxygen from the atmos-phere, for, without oxygen, our energy production would grind to a halt. It is true that we can consume energy, *for brief periods only*, by a built-in chemical 'borrowing' process which bypasses the *im-mediate* need for oxygen, but by so doing, we incur an 'oxygen debt' which must be repaid later. For example, the energy expended in a one hundred metre race is tremendous and this energy is consumed within a few seconds. In the few seconds it takes us to run one hundred metres, we simply do not have enough time to inhale all the oxygen we need in order to metabolise the amount of glucose required to produce the energy consumed in running the one hundred metres. Therefore, we 'borrow' the energy and we repay the 'oxygen debt' after the race by panting (i.e. breathing very deeply and rapidly), so that our oxygen intake will catch up with our energy consumption as quickly as possible. If we did not have this built-in chemical 'borrowing' process, we would not be able to run at all.

Our ability to absorb oxygen from the atmosphere depends upon the pressure of the oxygen within the atmosphere, which, in turn, depends upon the atmospheric pressure, and atmospheric pressure varies with altitude. As we ascend from sea level, the relative proportions of gases in the atmosphere remain the same, up to some 30 000 ft (9000 metres) above sea-level—e.g. oxygen remains at a constant 21 per cent of the atmosphere. However, with *increasing altitude*, there is *decreasing air density*, or (as some people prefer to put it) the air becomes 'more rarified'. In other words, there is less *total* air per cubic metre at 5000 ft than there is at sea level, and there is less *total* air at 10 000 ft than there is at 5000 ft and so on. Of course, this applies also to the oxygen in the air at different altitudes.

Concurrent with the decreasing amount of oxygen with increasing attitude is a decrease in *the pressure of the oxygen*, and it is upon this pressure that we depend for entry of oxygen into our lungs, whence it passes (because of a pressure gradient) into the bloodstream, and finally from the bloodstream into the body tissues. When the pressure of atmospheric oxygen is below a critical level we cannot absorb oxygen, and therefore we die from asphyxia. The critical altitude beyond which man cannot live without an oxygen mask is about 30 000 ft (9000 metres). This explains the fact that the tremendous achievement of climbing Mount Everest without breathing apparatus is *just* possible.

Hypoxia is the term given to oxygen-deprivation and, of course, its effects become increasingly apparent with increasing altitude. These effects include cyanosis, giddiness, vomiting, loss of self-criticism, disturbances of judgement and high-altitude respiration (see 'Respiration' in Part 11). The lowest altitude at which the effects of hypoxia become demonstrable is about 5000 ft (1500 metres) and this is called the threshold altitude for hypoxia. However, most fit people feel quite well at this altitude, and it is usually at altitudes in excess of 10 000 ft (3000 metres) that hypoxia problems begin in mountaineers. It is virtually impossible to predetermine who will be affected by hypoxia, or at what altitude. The only really effective treatment for hypoxia is to reduce altitude as quickly as possible. Obviously, hypoxia is not likely to be a problem in the British Isles where all the mountains are less than 5000 ft high; but *relative hypoxia* at 3000 ft (1000 metres) can add to the problems of injury and to exhaustion exposure (see below).

Having considered the relevant physiology, we can now consider the specific effects of exposure to extremes of temperature.

A. Exposure to heat

A person, who has been living in a cold or temperate climate, and who travels quickly to a tropical climate, requires time to acclimatise to the tropical heat. The minimum acclimatisation period is three weeks, but more time may be needed. Similarly, on return from the tropics to a temperate climate, it takes about three weeks to de-acclimatise.

Acclimatisation is effected by the thermoregulatory centre which *gradually* alters certain body functions. The two most important alterations are that:

a. the circulating volume of blood increases, which enhances heat loss by radiation and convection, and,

b. the sweating mechanism becomes more efficient (i.e. less sweat production is required in order to achieve the same heat loss), and this minimises the loss of water and salt as sweat.

However, *these readjustments of body functions take time.*

(1) Heat syncope

This occurs in the unacclimatised person. In response to tropical, or desert heat, the blood vessels in and under the skin dilate. This causes weakness, giddiness and fainting (i.e. syncope).

Treatment: Lie the victim down, raise his feet a little and protect him from direct sunlight. He will recover, as from a simple faint.

(2) Heat exhaustion (i.e. water depletion)

This is caused by failure to replace water lost as sweat. It affects the unacclimatised person more than the acclimatised, who sweats less than the unacclimatised. Increased water intake is the obvious answer. A daily intake of up to 7 litres (12 pints) may be required in the tropics.

(3) *Salt depletion*

Again, this occurs mainly in the unacclimatised. It is caused by increased loss of salt in sweat. It leads to exhaustion, nausea and even vomiting. A daily intake of between 15 and 25 grammes of salt may be needed to prevent salt depletion in the tropics. Even in temperate climates, many athletes take salt tables—e.g. tennis players during long matches.

(4) *Heat stroke*

Unlike the foregoing three conditions, heat stroke can cause death very rapidly. It can occur even in the acclimatised because of over-exertion.

The cause is complete failure of thermoregulation, whereas the three previous conditions occur as a result of normal, but excessive function of thermoregulation.

Effects. The body 'core' temperature rises rapidly to more than 40.6°C (105°F) There is a sudden onset of delirium, followed quickly by coma, and there is *complete absence of sweating*. If not treated promptly, this condition is fatal, because the temperature will rise rapidly, out of control, and the blood will boil (literally!)

Treatment of heat stroke

a. Ensure that the area is well-ventilated, or remove the victim to such an area.
b. *Cool the victim rapidly to below 39°C (102°F)* by *spraying* with cold water. A rectal thermometer is very helpful for this stage of treatment.
c. Below 39°C, cool the victim more slowly to prevent shut-down of skin vessels which may result in shock.

Heat waves in temperate climates can produce all four of these conditions because they last usually for a few days, and this is not enough time for acclimatisation. In one heat wave in the U.K., eight police cadets died whilst on a training walk over the hills. At autopsy, their blood was found to have boiled. Such was the effect of a heat wave in a normally temperate climate on eight, fit, young men.

Prevention of heat effects

This is really a matter of common sense. Nevertheless, I will list the necessary precautions:

a. Avoid, or avert, the direct heat from the sun, as much as possible.
b. Ensure adequate ventilation, whenever possible.
c. Ensure adequate fluid intake. (Not too much alcohol, which increases sweating.)
d. Ensure adequate salt intake.
e. Take a cool shower, whenever you think it necessary.
f. Avoid over-exertion. (*Exertion should be well below the normal maximum.*)

(5) Burns

This topic, alone, is sufficient to provide a medical debating society with enough arguments to keep its members occupied for a long time! There are many doctors who treat patients with burns. They all have their successes and yet their methods of classifying and of treating burns can, and do, vary tremendously. Therefore, I shall try to deal with this topic as simply and as briefly as possible.

When dealing with a patient with burns, we need to know (a) the age and sex of the patient, (b) what caused the burn, (c) the extent of the burn and (d) the depth of the burn.

a. The age and sex of the patient. These factors are important, because, in general after burns, younger people tend to be more resilient than older people; but it should be borne in mind that babies tolerate fluid loss very badly, and burns can be responsible for a great deal of fluid loss. Sex is important, because males have a relatively greater fluid reserve than females and are therefore able to tolerate fluid loss rather better than females.

b. The causative agent. Fire, boiling water and molten metals cause burns purely by destructive heat, which is self-limiting; but certain chemicals cause burns by chemical reactions with the body tissues; and some chemical burns require special remedies. The organic fluorides, for example, cause particularly nasty burns, which, if not treated properly, will increase in depth as the chemical continues to erode the body tissues. Therefore, it is important to ascertain the causative agent.

c. The extent of the burn (i.e. the amount, or percentage, of the surface area of the body which is affected by the burn). Here we find an astonishing amount of agreement amongst the burns experts! They all agree that the greater the surface area of the body covered by the burn, the greater the fluid loss the patient will (or is likely to) suffer. Also, most experts accept the 'rule of nines', which is a convenient, 'rule-of-thumb' method of dividing up the surface areas of the body. The 'rule of nines' divides the body into areas, each of which is nine per cent of the surface area of the body, or a multiple of nine per cent.

The exception to this rule is the one per cent attributed to the surface area of the external genitalia. Therefore, we have the areas as follows:

Surface area of	percentage
Head and neck	9
Right upper limb	9
Left upper limb	9
Front of trunk	18
Back of trunk	18
Right lower limb	18
Left lower limb	18
External genitalia	1
Total surface area	100

A patient with burns covering more than 20 per cent of the total surface area of the body (some would say more than 10 per cent) requires intravenous fluids. The greater the surface area involved by the burn, the greater the fluid loss expected and, therefore, the more urgent is the need to administer intravenous fluids.

d. The depth of the burn. This is where the experts start to disagree. The burn can affect the surface layer of the skin (epidermis) only, or it may affect deeper layers of the skin (the layers of the dermis), or the fatty tissue deep to the skin, or muscles and other structures at even deeper levels. The experts tend to classify the depth of burns as 'degrees', first degree burns always being the most superficial. According to which expert classifies burns, the degrees may be from first to third, first to fifth, first to seventh, or first to ninth. This variation of classification can be confusing for doctors, and even more so for First Aiders.

Fortunately, I have already solved the problem for First Aiders, because I have developed a very simple, but extremely practical classification of burns into two types—i.e. superficial and deep burns.

(i) *Superficial burns* are those in which the epidermis (the water-impervious layer of the skin) is damaged or destroyed. If it is damaged but remains in place covering the rest of the skin, serum oozes out from the deeper layers of the skin and blisters form. If the epidermis is destroyed (i.e. burned away from the rest of the skin), leaving the deeper layers (dermis) exposed, serum still oozes out and it drips onto the ground because there is no epidermis to contain it as blister fluid. A great deal of serum can be lost externally from such burns, depending upon their extent.

(ii) *Deep burns* are those in which the dermis and/or deeper layers (e.g. muscles) have been coagulated by the burn. Such coagulated tissues become water-impervious so that fluid is not lost externally from them, as with superficial burns. However, fluid loss does occur internally, deep to the coagulated layers which become separated from the healthy tissues by serum. If the burn is really deep and involves muscles, the blood vessels in the muscles are destroyed also, as are the red blood cells inside the blood vessels. If a lot of red blood cells are destroyed, the haemoglobin liberated from those red blood cells can block the filtering system of the kidneys, causing kidney failure.

So, purely from a practical point of view, superficial burns are those from which serum oozes outwards and either forms blisters or drips onto the ground. Deep burns are those where the deeper tissues are coagulated, so that serum cannot ooze outwards through them.

e. The treatment of burns. Now this is where expert opinion really diversifies, and has done so for many years. There are just about as many different burns regimes as there are consultants who treat burns; but, fortunately for the first aider, the consultants deal with the *definitive* treatment of burns—i.e. the hospital in-patient and out-patient treatment of burns—whereas the first aider's concern is the first aid treatment of burns. This 'lets me off the hook' nicely, because, as far as definitive treatment is concerned, I can say, quite simply, that the choice of definitive treatment is entirely up to the particular consultant in the particular hospital in which the burned patient is being treated. However, I think that most consultants would agree with the following points on the first aid treatment of burns:

(i) *Immediate actions*

(a) Heat burns—i.e. those caused purely by heat (eg. from fire, boiling water, hot metal, or burning petrol)—should be immersed in cold water, immediately after the burn has occurred. This minimises the total tissue damage. If the burns cover extensive areas (e.g. 60–80 per cent of the body), immersion in a *cool* bath is advisable, but not a cold bath since this may worsen shock.

(b) Cold burns (e.g. from carbon dioxide snow) should, for similar reasons, be immersed in warm water.

(c) Chemical burns should, ideally, be treated immediately with the specific chemical antidote, but if this is not possible, the alternative is to irrigate the burn *liberally* with water.

(ii) *Subsequent actions*

(a) DO NOT pull off anything which is adherent to the surface of the wound—e.g. clothing, toffee, jam, tar, or metal—since this may cause unnecessary damage to the wound.

(b) DO NOT put anything onto the surface of the burn which will colour it (e.g. Acriflavine causes a yellow stain). Colouring agents alter the true appearance of the burn and this makes life difficult for the doctor in the accident unit.

(c) The surface of the burn should be covered with a clean (preferably sterile), non-fluffy and, ideally, non-adherent dressing. For the purpose of a *Short* journey to hospital, dampened gauze forms a reasonably non-adherent dressing.

(d) Bandage the dressing *firmly*, to minimise fluid loss, especially from superficial burns; but ensure that the bandage is *not tight*, so that it will not impair the circulation in, or near, the affected part.

(e) For extensive burns, intravenous fluids should be commenced as soon as possible. Ideally, this should be done *before* transporting the patient to hospital.

(f) Strong pain-killers, such as morphine and papaveretum, may be necessary, especially for extensive superficial burns which can be extremely painful, since the loss of the epidermis tends to leave bared pain-fibres in the surface of the wound. Deep burns often destroy the pain-fibres in the dermis and, therefore, after the initial pain during burning, the patient may not feel much pain at all.

(g) Transport the patient to hospital as soon as possible, but please ensure that the patient's journey is as comfortable as possible. He should be transported in the position which he finds most comfortable. The head-down position is useful for shocked patients. Remember that the pain and fluid loss of burns cause shock, and that rough transportation aggravates shock.

B. Exposure to cold

This brings us to the hypothermias and frostbite.

(1) *Baby hypothermia*

This results from inadequate energy production, or excessive heat loss, or a combination of the two.

    a. Inadequate energy production results from inadequate food intake or absorption. Inadequate food intake is usually an effect of poverty rather than of parental neglect. Inadequate absorption of food products can be caused by numerous diseases, especially gastroenteritis, in which vomiting and diarrhoea cause loss of food products and a great deal of fluid. Vomiting often accompanies a high temperature in babies whatever the reason for the high temperature (e.g. kidney infections; pneumonia).

    b. Excessive heat loss can be caused by inadequate insulation (i.e. clothing), a very cold environment, or a combination of the two. Here, again, disease can play a part, because, during infections, the metabolic rate of the baby increases in order to combat the invading organism. This increase in metabolism causes the temperature to rise. Since a baby's heat conservation mechanism is less well developed than that of an adult, the greater the heat production, the greater the heat loss.

    Prevention: This is rather obvious, but:

a. Ensure adequate food intake, at appropriate intervals, for the baby.
b. Ensure that the baby has adequate clothing and a sufficiently warm environment.
c. Sterilise the baby's feeding utensils.
d. Keep sources of infection away from the baby (*especially* doting relatives with 'stinking' colds!)

    Treatment.   Because of their low energy reserves, babies can become hypothermic quite quickly, and they do not accumulate harmful by-products of metabolism in quantities comparable to those which can accumulate in adults. Therefore, the treatment is to *rewarm babies quickly* because they can tolerate it. Hot water bottles can be a very useful first aid measure, but *DON'T* let them burn the baby. Place a blanket between the hot water bottles and the baby to avoid direct contact and burns.

(2) *Hypothermia of the elderly*

Frail, elderly people need extra clothes and an external heat source (e.g. a fire) in order to keep warm. If such a person falls in the home and cannot get up again, then he will become cold unless he happens to have fallen near to the heat source. Hypertension, pneumonia or an accident may account for the fall, but if the person cannot get up (e.g. because of a fractured neck of femur or a stroke), hypothermia is highly likely to ensue, particularly when the elderly person lives alone. In the U.K., hypothermia of the elderly can occur even in summer, though it usually occurs in winter.

Prevention.   A great deal of literature on the subject of prevention of hypothermia in the elderly exists already. For present purposes, I must deal with it briefly, by stating that the important features of prevention can be summed up in one word—'Care'. If enough care is exercised by enough people (relatives, friends, neighbours, members of the Health Services and members of the Social Services), then a great deal of hypothermia of the elderly can be prevented.

Treatment.   This consists of *gradual re-warming*. The elderly hypothermic person has usually been lying on the floor for a number of hours, becoming increasingly cold, and therefore has had time to accumulate harmful by-products of metabolism by the time he is found. Rapid re-warming would improve the circulation too quickly, and this would mobilise too many harmful by-products of metabolism too quickly. The brain would then receive a lethal dose of these by-products. So, remember, *rapid re-warming of elderly hypothermic patients is lethal*.

As a first aid measure, a space blanket' (or even wrapping the patient in baking foil) can be useful in preventing further heat loss. In hospital, the patient is allowed to re-warm gradually, in bed under blankets and in a warm (*but not hot*) room. Ideally, hot water bottles should not be necessary if the room temperature is adequate; but if they have to be used (e.g. because of a failure in the central heating system), they should be placed around the patient and on top of the blankets. The patient should not be able to feel the hot water bottles through the blankets and must *NEVER* be allowed to come into direct contact with hot water bottles since this can prove lethal, or (at best) can burn the patient's skin.

(3) Immersion hypothermia

This occurs, when someone falls into very cold water, the temperature of the water being so low that the body loses heat to the water very rapidly by direct conduction. For instance, a man in ordinary clothing who falls into the North Sea (the sea between Scotland and Norway), has a life expectancy of about ten minutes, in summer, and only four minutes, in winter. If the same man were to fall into the Arctic Ocean, then his life expectancy (in winter or summer) would be an agonising two minutes, during which time his body heat would be drawn out of him, as if by strong magnetism, and death would bring a welcome relief to his agony. Immersion hypothermia can occur at any age, but it occurs most commonly in seafarers and yachtsmen who are usually in the teenager-to-middle-aged range. However, immersion hypothermia can occur in walkers of any age who fall into cold lakes and rivers. Snow avalanche victims suffer immersion hypothermia from sudden immersion in snow.

Prevention.   (Dare I say it?) Don't fall into cold water! If entering very cold water deliberately, wear the correct protective attire.

Treatment.   *Rapid re-warming* is the treatment of choice because the immersion has caused rapid cooling and there has been insufficient time for toxic by-products of metabolism to accumulate in the body. *If the person can summon up the energy*, he should be encouraged to run around so that he will increase his heat production by consuming energy. His skin should be dried as quickly as possible, and cold wet clothing should be replaced by dry clothing in abundance. On land, a tent should be erected and, if possible, a fire lit so that he can relax in warmth, protected from wind-chill effect after his energy-consuming 'warm-up'. Food and hot drinks will then be most welcome.

If the person is so cold that he cannot summon up the energy to run around, he may well have to be treated as for Exhaustion exposure (see below), unless a hot bath is readily available which is often the case in ships. *The hot bath treatment* consists of immersing the rescued victim (with the exception of his nose and mouth, of course) in a bath of water at 45°C (113°F). This will restore the victim of immersion hypothermia to warmth, health and comfort quite quickly and safely; *but it must NEVER be used to treat a victim of exhaustion exposure.*

(4) *Exhaustion exposure* (also known as 'Mountain hypothermia')

The term 'Exhaustion exposure' describes this condition concisely, because it consists of exhaustion, both physical and mental, in combination with exposure to cold weather. It occurs commonly in fell-walkers and mountaineers. Hence, the alternative name of 'Mountain hypothermia'. The simple terms, 'exposure' and 'hypothermia', were used formerly to describe this condition, but they were such vague terms that they have now been abandoned by the vast majority of mountain rescue teams. No matter which term is preferred, this condition is a serious one because *it can prove fatal within two hours of onset* if not dealt with promptly and correctly.

Contributing factors. These are numerous, but they can be divided into two basic groups:

a. *Environmental factors*
  (i) *Ambient air temperature* (i.e. the temperature of the surrounding air). If the ambient air temperature is low, then soil, shale, scree, rocks and crag faces become cool too. Therefore, body heat can be lost by radiation to the air and by conduction through contact with cold surfaces. These effects are countered by a shut-down of the skin blood vessels and the skin feels cold. In fact, the temperature difference between the body 'core' and the body 'shell' may be quite considerable, but this is no great detriment, provided that the body 'core' temperature remains healthy and that frostbite does not occur.
  (ii) *Wind-chill effect.* In cold weather, the wind enhances the effect of the ambient air temperature by adding convection heat-loss to the body's problems. For a given ambient air temperature, an increase in wind velocity will produce an increase in cooling of the body surface and *this occurs on a logarithmic scale.*

For example, a wind velocity of 10 m.p.h. (18 (18 km.p.h.) is *twice* as great as a wind velocity of 5 m.p.h. (9 km.p.h.) Yet, the 10 m.p.h. wind will exert about *four times* as much cooling effect as the 5 m.p.h. wind. Similarly, a 20 m.p.h. wind will exert about four times the cooling effect of the 10 m.p.h. wind, and so on. Given an ambient temperature of 0°C (32°F) and zero wind velocity, a man dressed only in summer clothing could survive for some considerable time, but the same man could tolerate 0°C and a

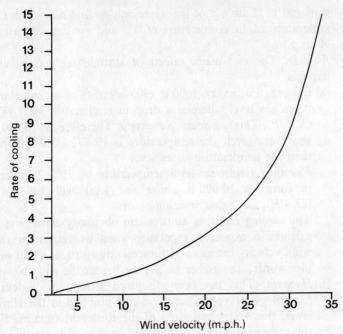

Fig. 27

wind velocity of 30 m.p.h. (54 km.p.h.) for only a few minutes before being forced to shiver violently to maintain his body 'core'
temperature.

(iii) *Rain, mist and cloud.* Rain can fall onto the surface of the body,
whilst mist and cloud can condense on the body surface. *Snow*
can also melt on the body surface. All of these factors produce
a wet body surface, from which heat can be lost by evaporation. (If moisture evaporates from a cagoule, then the cagoule
loses heat, too.) Thus, there is an evaporative heat-loss problem, which is also enhanced by wind velocity, *again on a logarithmic scale,* and the wind velocity effect is even greater when
we emerge from rain, mist or cloud into clear air, because
evaporation takes place more easily in clear air than in rainy,
misty, foggy and cloudy atmospheres. Under conditions of
0°C, a wind velocity of 30 m.p.h. and having just emerged
from cloud into clear air, our man in summer clothing would
die, without almost immediate shelter and warmth. He could
expect a similar fate if he fell into ice-cold water and then

managed to climb out of the water only to find himself in the same ambient air temperature of 0°C and a wind velocity of 30 m.p.h.

(iv) *Altitude*. The two major effects of altitude are cooling and hypoxia.

(a) *Cooling*. For every 1000 ft (305 metres) of ascent above mean sea level, there is a drop in temperature of 1.98°C (3.56°F). *This is a direct relationship*. Therefore, at 10 000 ft above sea level, the temperature is 19.8°C (35.6°F) *lower* than the temperature at sea level.

Example: Given sea-level temperature of 15°C, the temperature at 10 000 ft above sea level will be—4.8°C (23.4°F), i.e. below freezing point.

The cooling effect of altitude can obviously contribute to exhaustion exposure, especially when we remember that wind velocity increases with increasing altitude; or, in simpler words, 'the higher we go, the harder the wind blows'.

(b) *Hypoxia*. This has been discussed already in 'Relevant physiology'. Hypoxia can be a real problem in the Himalayas, the Andes and parts of the Rocky Mountains. For this reason, and because giddiness, nausea and vomiting are such common symptoms of hypoxia, mountaineers refer to the symptoms and signs of hypoxia as 'mountain sickness'. In the U.K., hypoxia is rarely, if ever, a problem for mountaineers, but *relative hypoxia* (at, say 3000 ft) can constitute an aggravating factor in exhaustion exposure, especially in a person who is immobilised because of an injury, and who has lost blood (see 'Personal factors' (viii), below).

b. *Personal factors*—These are numerous and include the following:

(i) *Personal fitness*. This is an obvious factor. *Really* fit people usually stay that way!

(ii) *Illness*. This affects the level of personal fitness adversely.

(iii) *Diet*. Before a long walk, a walker should have a nutritious food and fluid intake. He should take ample food and fluid with him for the journey.

(iv) *Clothes*. These should include waterproofs (which are also windproof!), and extra sweaters. *NEVER* start a walk overclothed, because this causes overheating and discomfort which lead rapidly to fatigue. Feeling a little chilly is the ideal way to set out for a long walk.

(v) *Sleep*. Those who have a good sleep before a walk, are less likely to become fatigued than those who sleep badly.

(vi) *Psychological factors*. These are potentially multitudinous. They range from lack of self-confidence to worrying about a sick relative!

(vii) *Drugs*. Many drugs can slow the thought processes and hence the reaction time of a person. They include antihistamines (often used by hay fever sufferers), tranquillisers, sedatives, antidepressants and hypnotics. The effects of these drugs on the brain is increased by altitude (because of hypoxia, or even relative hypoxia). If exhaustion exposure commences, these drugs will increase the rate of progress of the effects of exhaustion exposure on the brain (see below).

(viii) *Immobilisation*. In walkers and climbers, the commonest cause of this is injury, especially injury to a lower limb or to the spine. Whilst lying on the ground, a walker's activity (and, therefore, heat production) is decreased, and there can be considerable conductive heat-loss if he is not insulated adequately from the ground.

(ix) *Age factor*. Young adults and middle-aged people succumb to exhaustion exposure less than do teenagers. This is largely due to metabolic factors, but, no doubt, experience plays a part, too.

(x) *Boots*. I mention these last, though they are by no means the least important in the list. Apart from insulating our feet from cold ground and water, our boots should provide our feet with support and *comfort*. To have sore feet after walking five miles, with the prospect of another ten or fifteen miles ahead, can be very demoralising indeed. Remember that *your boots can be your best friends, or your worst enemies!*

Effects of exhaustion exposure

The basic effect of exhaustion exposure is that the body 'core' begins to cool *and continues to cool*. This is reflected in *further* cooling of the already cold body 'shell', notably the skin, and this provides us with a good rule-of-thumb method of early diagnosis of the condition (see below). The cooling of the body 'core' includes cooling of the blood in the body 'core', and this has internal effects, particularly on the brain, heart, liver, muscles, and respiration.

(i) *The brain* is affected first. Initially, there is a depression of mood, and the sufferer feels and looks unhappy. This is followed by irritability, confusion, blurred vision, hallucinations, and loss of co-ordination of physical activity. Nausea and vomiting are quite common, too. Eventually unconsciousness supervenes.

(ii) *The heart* becomes less efficient. The circulatory rate declines, and blood tends to 'pool' in the limbs, where it becomes increasingly contaminated by the harmful by-products of metabolism.

(iii) *The liver* becomes less efficient too. There is progressive impairment of its ability to release stored food-products into the bloodstream and of its ability to detoxify the harmful by-products of metabolism.

(iv) *The muscles* become progressively weaker and their actions become uncoordinated. With progressive cooling of the body, *shivering ceases*. Finally, the muscles become too weak to support the sufferer, who collapses and loses consciousness rapidly. *If not treated adequately, he will die within two hours.*

(v) *Respiration* declines too, in both rate and volume.

Prevention of exhaustion exposure lies in avoiding, or countering, the contributory factors.

Early recognition of exhaustion exposure. This is important. The sooner it is recognised, the better for everyone in the party. Early recognition depends on astute observation and a 'rule-of-thumb' assessment of the sufferer's temperature, which is surprisingly accurate.

a. *Astute observation.* If you are on the hill and you notice that one of your party is looking pale and miserable, observe his gait. If he steps a little falteringly, or 'not quite as positively as he might', then your suspicions should be aroused and you should assess his temperature by:

b. *'Rule-of-thumb' temperature assessment.* Remove a glove and expose your hand to the cold for a few minutes until your fingers feel definitely cold to your own forehead. Now, place the temperature-sensitive skin of your fingers (i.e. that on the back of the *middle* bone of each finger) against the forehead of the suspect. If his forehead feels cold to your already-cold fingers, then he has begun to suffer from exhaustion exposure, and you should commence treatment *at once*. I have used this test a number of times and have found it remarkably accurate.

Treatment. The objectives of treatment are:

a. *To prevent further heat loss.* Elimination of wind-chill effect and insulation of the sufferer from the ground are the important measures here. Rucksacks can provide good, temporary insulation from the ground whilst a tent is being erected to provide protection from the wind. When the tent has been erected, a number of unrolled sleeping bags, one on top of the other, provide good ground-insulation inside the tent. (N.B. The sewn-in groundsheet of a tent provides dryness, but *not* insulation against heat-loss.) Obviously, the sufferer should be covered, too.

b. *To avoid shunting toxic blood from the limbs to the body 'core', which could prove fatal.* Undue alteration of the sufferer's posture and undue movements of his limbs can cause the highly toxic, cold blood of the body 'shell' to move to the body 'core' and displace its relatively warm and less toxic blood which will then be shunted into the body 'shell'. The unconscious sufferer already has quite enough toxic by-products of metabolism in his body core, otherwise he would not be unconscious, and he needs a decrease in them, not an increase! Therefore:

  (i) Whatever the *posture* of the sufferer who is unconscious when found, it should be maintained until he regains consciousness (provided that it is compatible with breathing, of course). The posture, when found, should be maintained whilst he is being carried into the tent and whilst he is warming in the tent.

  (ii) WET CLOTHING MUST NOT BE REMOVED FROM THE UNCONSCIOUS EXHAUSTION EXPOSURE SUFFERER UNTIL CONSCIOUSNESS HAS BEEN FULLY RE-ESTABLISHED.

c. *To re-warm the sufferer GRADUALLY.* In this condition the body needs time to return to normal function. In particular, the liver needs time to recover so that it can deal with the accumulated toxic by-products of metabolism. Gradual re-warming can be achieved by packing the tent with as many people as possible. This increases the air temperature inside the tent quite quickly, but to a level which will not cause rapid re-heating of the sufferer. It has the additional advantage that other members of the party are protected from wind-chill as well as the sufferer! Some people prefer to put someone into a casualty bag with the sufferer to act as a 'human hot water bottle'. I call this the 'Eskimo treatment' because Eskimos have used it successfully for centuries. When the sufferer regains consciousness fully (usually within two hours), he should have dry clothing substituted for wet and he should be given food and warm (*not hot*) drinks. Given time to recover, most exhaustion exposure sufferers should become fit enough to walk off the hill, under escort, provided that they have no physical injuries, *and this will restore their self-confidence*. This is the *ideal* ultimate objective in the treatment of exhaustion exposure. There is nothing more demoralising for a walker than to start out on a walk and to finish up being carried off the hill on a stretcher without having sustained any physical injury.

However, it is not always possible to achieve ideal objectives. Some exhaustion exposure sufferers who have been *deeply* hypothermic, may remain weak for a few days after recovery. Also, the vast majority of Mountain Rescue personnel in the U.K. are unpaid volunteers, and they cannot afford to ignore their own personal schedules, particularly their work schedules. Therefore, when the exhaustion exposure sufferer has regained consciousness, and when his general condition is adequately stabilised, he can be carried off the hill, if he is still weak. This is a reasonable compromise between expediency and the time factor which would be required in order to achieve the ideal ultimate objective.

If exhaustion exposure is recognised early, it may be sufficient to use large rocks or the foot of a crag as improvised protection from the wind, and to huddle round the sufferer and allow him food, warm drinks and rest. *But*, please remember to insulate him from the ground and rocks and give him as much extra clothing as possible, ensuring that the outermost layer is windproof and waterproof. When he has re-warmed, take a route off the hill which is as short and safe as possible.

Comments

(i) *The hot bath treatment is at least potentially lethal for exhaustion exposure sufferers.* (In any case, there are no hot baths readily available on mountains!)

(ii) It may happen that a walker falls into a cold lake, gets out, cools very rapidly and becomes unconscious before he is found. The golden rule is that, *if there is any doubt as to the diagnosis* (i.e. immersion hypothermia or exhaustion exposure) *treat as for exhaustion exposure*.

(iii) Occasionally, exhaustion exposure victims have been found apparently dead, but, on being re-warmed, they have recovered, *even though their corneal reflexes were absent* when they were found. (See Diagnosis of death.) Therefore, *it is impera-*

tive to re-warm such people for up to two hours. If, after re-warming, their corneal reflexes are still absent, then they may be pronounced dead.

(iv) For further reading on the subject of exhaustion exposure, I can do no better than refer you to a two-part article on the subject which was published in the September and October (1977) editions of the magazine *Climber and Rambler*. It is entitled, 'Exhaustion exposure', and was written by Dr James Ogilvy, Medical Officer to the Patterdale Mountain Rescue Team in the Lake District of England. *It is an authoritative article based on Dr Ogilvy's experience, and I recommend it most strongly.* For further details, see page 99.

(5) *Frostbite*

In this condition, the circulation in the affected part stops altogether and the fluid inside the cells of the affected part freezes. The toes, fingers and nose are most commonly affected, but other parts of the body may be affected.

Symptoms. These vary. Coldness, then tingling progressing to painfulness, may be felt. On the other hand, numbness may be the only symptom, or there may be a complete absence of symptoms.

Signs:

(i) *Early* on, the affected part is white and waxy, surrounded by a red zone.

(ii) *Later*, the affected part becomes purplish, or bluish.

(iii) *Finally*, the affected part becomes black, indicating tissue death (i.e. gangrene.)

The recommended treatment is rapid re-warming as soon as possible by one of the following methods:

(i) Immerse the affected part in water at 45°C (113°F), or

(ii) Warm the affected part in the armput or groin, or

(iii) Massage *GENTLY*

N.B. (i) *NEVER* rub vigorously with snow or ice.

(ii) If the affected part is black (i.e. dead), it is too late to re-warm it. It should be kept as dry as possible. A demarcation layer will form between the living tissue and the gangrenous tissue, and this will gradually cut off the living from the gangrenous tissue. Eventually, the gangrenous tissue will drop off, having been rejected by the body.

(iii) If gangrenous tissue becomes soggy, it is in great danger of becoming infected, and the infecting organisms may penetrate the demarcation layer. The infection can, then, spread to the rest of the limb or even to the rest of the body, and may prove fatal. THEREFORE, GANGREN-OUS TISSUE MUST BE KEPT DRY!

C. Exposure to altitude

'*Mountain sickness*' (*acute mountain sickness*) is a term used by moun-taineers to describe illness which results from rapid ascent to high altitudes (i.e. to above 10 000 ft above sea level). The occurrence of acute mountain sickness cannot be predicted accurately for any one person, but, in general, the least fit people are the ones most likely to suffer it.

One classification of acute mountain sickness is that of a benign form and three malignant forms of acute mountain sickness, thus:

(i) Benign acute mountain sickness

Some, or all of the following symptoms occur: headache, nausea, loss of appetite, vomiting, weakness, insomnia, light-headedness and discomfort in the chest. These symptoms are probably caused by a *combination of hypoxia and prolonged exposure to reduced atmos-pheric pressure*. The symptoms are very similar to those of hypoxia. Yet the discomfort in the chest is as described by aviators who suf-fer *decompression sickness*, the threshold altitude for which is 18 000 ft (5500 metres). A combination of hypoxia with prolonged exposure to reduced atmospheric pressure could well explain the three types of malignant acute mountain sickness.

(ii) Malignant acute mountain sickness

a. *Cerebral acute mountain sickness.* This causes loss of physical co-ordination (ataxia), irritability, abnormal behaviour, drowsiness, hallucinations, coma and incontinence of urine.
b. *Pulmonary acute mountain sickness.* This causes breathlessness at rest, cough, white frothy sputum and cyanosis. The heart rate is rapid and there are crepitations (high-pitched, bubbling sounds) at the bases of the lungs (i.e. at the back of the chest, just above the kidneys).
c. *Mixed forms of acute mountain sickness.* These combine features of the cerebral and pulmonary types.
   Treatment. For the malignant forms of acute mountain sickness,

descent to a lower altitude is absolutely essential, otherwise death will ensue. For the benign form, it is apparently sufficient for most people to rest at the same altitude in order to recover; but if the illness progresses towards one of the malignant forms, then descent becomes mandatory. Certainly, no further ascent should be made until the sufferer feels quite well again. If in any doubt about the sufferer's rate of recovery, or ability to recover, from benign acute mountain sickness, let the golden rule be, '*If in doubt, descent*'.

Prevention

a. A high standard of personal fitness is the most important preventative factor.
b. Avoid taking drugs, which may cause drowsiness. At high altitudes, these drugs have increased cerebral effects. There is a whole host of such drugs, and *alcohol* is included in the list!
c. There is good evidence that Acetazolamide (Diamox), taken *once* daily, after breakfast, in the form of a slow-release 500 mg sustet, helps to prevent acute mountain sickness.

SUGGESTED FURTHER READING

(1) Dr James Ogilvie—'Exhaustion exposure'—a two part article produced in the September and October, 1977, editions of the magazine, *Climber and Rambler*. Copies of this article can be obtained from the publishers, Holmes McDougall Ltd, Allander House, Leith Walk, Edinburgh, Scotland.
(2) Dr J.G. Dickinson—'Terminology and classification of acute mountain sickness'. A very readable and interesting article published in the *British Medical Journal* of 11th September 1982 (Volume 285, pages 720 and 721). Again, this is *highly recommended reading*, because it is based on the personal experience of the author who is Consultant Physician at Shanta Bhawan Hospital, Katmandu, Nepal. Copies of this article may be obtained from the British Medical Association B.M.A. House, Tavistock square, London WCiH 9JR, England.
(3) Alfred Gregory—'Diamox'—an interesting, short article, published in the magazine, *Climber and Rambler*, September 1982 edition. Copies may be obtained from the publishers, Holmes McDougall Ltd, Allander House, Leith Walk, Edinburgh, Scotland.
(4) J.G. Dickinson 1972 Postgrad. Med. J., 55, 454–8.

4. ELECTRIC SHOCK

This may cause unconsciousness (see 'infarct' below).

'I'

1. INJURY TO THE HEAD

This is dealt with later (see *Head injuries*).

2. INFARCT OR CORONARY THROMBOSIS

In this condition the patient complains typically of a severe tight or crushing pain in the front of the chest and there may also be pain down the left arm, or even down both arms. Occasionally there may be pain in the front of the neck, but this is far more common in angina. The pain is so severe that the patient is often pale and sweating, and he may vomit. He may collapse and become unconscious because of heart failure. Sometimes, a person who suffers a massive coronary thrombosis may just collapse and become unconscious, without even complaining of pain. External cardiac massage has been advocated in the past but on more than one occasion it has done the patient more harm than good.

In one case, a woman who collapsed was treated with external cardiac massage, but died. A post mortem examination revealed fractured ribs, lacerations to the liver and a rupture of the diaphragm, with gross bleeding into the abdomen, which was considered to be the cause of death. The moral from this is 'Either do it right, or just do not do it'. I, myself, have tried to revive people by cardiac massage (external *and internal*), when they have collapsed after coronaries. So far, my failure rate is 100 per cent! In other words, external cardiac massage is most unlikely to restart a heart which has stopped because of a coronary. It is far more likely to be successful after electric shock, but even then, another electric shock from a defibrillator is far more likely to be successful. The reason for this is that, after an electric shock the heart muscle itself is not damaged, but it has lost its ability to contract in a properly co-ordinated fashion. A coronary thrombosis causes the death of a part of the heart muscle, and therefore the dead part of the heart muscle is unable to contract, no matter what you do to it.

Those people who are revived by external cardiac massage after a coronary thrombosis are usually found to have had a small infarct, which has affected the heart's ability to contract in a co-ordinated fashion (cf. electric shock). The most important thing is to confirm the diagnosis of cardiac arrest, *before* embarking upon external cardiac massage. The diagnosis is confirmed by:

a. inability to feel a pulse, and
b. inability to hear a heartbeat.

If external cardiac massage has been continued for ten minutes, and if the pulse cannot be felt, nor the heartbeat heard, then further cardiac massage will prove useless.

'O'

OVERDOSE (another aspect of Toxicology)

Opiates are the derivatives of opium, which comes from the opium poppy. They include Morphine, Pethidine, Codeine, Papaveretum, ('Omnopon') and Diamorphine ('Heroin'). Nowadays, there are many other drugs which, in overdose, can cause unconsciousness. These newer drugs are members of the two groups known as Tranquillisers and Antidepressants and they are too numerous to list here (apart from which, I would not wish to incur the wrath of any particular drug firm!) There is also the group of drugs known as Barbiturates. These have been on the market for many years.

A person who has taken an overdose of a drug first of all becomes drowsy but rouseable. Later he becomes unrouseable but irritable. Then he becomes unresponsive, and during this stage the pupils vary in size individually. At one moment the right pupil may be larger than the left, and the next moment the reverse may be the case. Depending on how much of the drug has been absorbed into the bloodstream, the person may die, or he may survive. If he survives, he will wake up with an almighty 'hangover'!

'U'

Uraemia

This is a condition in which there is a great build-up of urea in the blood. It occurs because the kidneys are so badly diseased that they are unable to perform their normal function. If a person is so uraemic that he becomes unconscious, then the outlook is very grave indeed. As a First Aider you are most unlikely to see this condition, because the patient will probably have been ill in bed for a long time.

'3Ds'

1. Diabetes mellitus

This should be no stranger to anyone, these days. I will simply remind you that there are two types of coma, which may occur in diabetes:

(a) Hypoglycaemia (Insulin coma). It is caused either by not eating after a normal dose of insulin, or by an accidental overdose of insulin and it results in a low blood sugar. The patient becomes pale, cold and clammy, and his pulse becomes increasingly slower and weaker. If you reach him before he becomes unconscious, try to give him something to eat, preferably sugar or glucose. If he is unconscious already, he should be taken to hospital, because he needs to have glucose injected into a vein.

(b) Hyperglycaemia (Ketotic coma). In this condition, the diabetes is out of control and the blood sugar is very high, hence the name *hyper*glycaemia (Hyper = above. Hypo = below). However, I must stress that it is NOT the increased blood sugar which is responsible for the coma. It is the build-up of ketones which does the damage. In diabetes mellitus, the patient cannot complete the breakdown of glucose into carbon dioxide and water. Instead, he reaches only the half-way stage in the breakdown process. He manages to break down each glucose molecule into two ketone molecules and is then unable to proceed any further. Since he has obtained much less energy from one glucose molecule than the normal person would, he continues his quest for further energy by liberating into his bloodstream far more glucose than the normal person would, and again the glucose is broken down only as far as the ketone stage, which is as far as the diabetic can go. Now, these ketones are poisonous to the human body. So, if they can be broken down into the relatively harmless carbon dioxide and water—as happens in the normal person—then all is well. However, the diabetic *cannot* break them down. Instead he builds up a concentration within himself until a very dangerous level is reached, at which stage he goes into coma. If he is not treated promptly, he will die. So remember, it is the ketones which do the damage, not the glucose. For this reason *hyperglycaemic coma* is often referred to as *ketotic coma*.

The person in ketotic coma has a dry, flushed face, a rapid, bounding pulse and deep, rapid respiration. The sweet-smelling breath is due to the ketones, which he is trying desperately to exhale, just as a normal person would exhale carbon dioxide. He must be admitted to hospital so that:

a. his life can be saved and,

b. his treatment can be stabilised before he is allowed to go home.

Some diagnostic confusion may arise from the fact that before unconsciousness supervenes the patient may become agitated, even aggressive, and this produces a marked increase in the rates and volumes of both pulse and respiration. In effect, this is Stage 2

Table 1 Comparison of the signs of established insulin and ketotic comas

Signs	Insulin coma	Ketotic coma
face	pale, cold and clammy	dry and flushed
pulse rate	reduced	increased
pulse volume	weak	bounding
respiratory rate	reduced	increased
respiratory volume	shallow	deep

Anaesthesia (see 'Classical stages of anaesthesia'). Yet, once the coma is *established*, then:

(i) the clinical diagnosis becomes clear and,

(ii) *un*treated, the patient has a life expectancy of only about two hours. So, seek medical assistance, quickly!

If you compare the signs of *established* hypoglycaemic and ketotic comas, you will see that the facial appearances are different, pulse rate and volume are different and so are the respiratory rate and volume. Therefore, normally, you should have little difficulty in distinguishing one from the other.

However, if you find a diabetic who is drowsy (i.e. in a pre-comatose condition) and if there is any doubt in your mind at all as to which kind of coma he is going into, then *make him eat sugar*, as much as possible. As I have said already sugar, or glucose, does no harm. Therefore, if he is going into hypoglycaemic coma, the sugar will revive him. If he is going into ketotic coma, sugar will not revive him, though it will do him no harm. This is the way to prove your diagnosis, one way or the other, and perhaps to revive the patient. So, NEVER BE AFRAID TO GIVE SUGAR TO A DIABETIC.

2. DRUNK (i.e. alcohol intoxication; yet another aspect of toxicology).

This speaks for itself! Since alcohol is a drug of intoxication it could have been included under Overdose, but it just happens to be convenient to use as the second of the '3 Ds'. Otherwise there would only be 2 Ds.

The signs are very similar to those of the overdose. Alcohol first causes a slight slowing of mental processes. Then it produces elation and the person appears more alert, and may increase the speed of speech, writing etc. However, at the same time, the *accuracy* (of speech writing, driving, typing etc.) is *decreased*. Later, speech and actions become progressively slower, and unconsciousness supervenes. The 'give-away' sign is, of course, the smell of alcohol on the breath. Having said that, it should be pointed out that a drunken man may collapse because of a stroke, coronary thrombosis, epilepsy, etc.

3. DEAD (AND DIAGNOSIS OF DEATH)

Death is death, or is it? Death can be defined in many ways, none of which is complete and accurate in itself. When a person has ceased to be capable of functioning as an independent individual, the cells of the body continue to function for a number of hours afterwards, until each cell, in its own time, gradually grinds to a halt. Therefore, death is extremely difficult, if not impossible, to define. It is much easier to accept that death is death and that we know of certain signs, which enable us to make a diagnosis of death. I know that death is a diagnosis which First Aiders are reluctant to make. Perhaps this is because it is so final, and they do not wish to declare someone dead, who may be alive. However, it is important to be able to make this diagnosis, especially when dealing with mass casualties, when priority of evacuation becomes so vital. Those in the worst condition must be evacuated first, if you are to save the maximum number of lives possible. Obviously you would not send a dead person to a mortuary in preference to sending a living person to hospital. Also, you would send a conscious person with multiple injuries away first, in preference to an unconscious person already displaying Cheyne-Stokes respiration whose chances are nil. The ethics of priority of evacuation in peacetime are debatable, but the object should be to save as many recoverable people as possible and not to endanger the recoverable lives by giving priority of evacuation to the irrecoverable. The 'brain scanner' is used now in hospitals, together with the electroencephalograph, to detect brain death; but first aiders can hardly be expected to carry pocket-sized brain scanners! So let us now consider the clinical signs which assist us to make a diagnosis of death.

a. Early signs of death

If you come across a dead man soon after death then usually you will find that he is motionless, but on occasions, there may be spontaneous unco-ordinated twitching movements, especially if death has been caused by violent crush-injury to the head. These movements last for only a few minutes. Electric shock may cause an immediate stiffening of all the muscles of the body, known as Cadaveric Spasm. Usually however, the limbs are found to be quite flaccid (i.e. floppy). The eyes are fixed and staring, with the pupils fixed, dilated and unresponsive to light. Both the lash reflex and the corneal reflex are absent (see notes 1 and 2 below). The pulses are absent (radial, carotid and femoral), as is the heartbeat. Chest movement is absent and the 'mirror-sign' is negative (see note 3). If you place your ear to his chest, you will not hear any breath sounds, but be careful not to press on the chest, or you may expel air and this would give you the false impression that he is alive! About twenty minutes after the circulation has ceased, the corneae (the 'windows' of the eyes) become glazed and opaque. This is because of lack of lubrication of the corneae by tears, which have ceased to be produced by the tear glands.

Explanatory notes

(i) *Lash reflex*

If you touch your own, or someone else's eyelash, it causes the eyelids to blink. This is the lash reflex.

(ii) *Corneal reflex*

CAREFUL! This is very painful to the conscious person. If you touch the cornea it will cause a sustained blink. Just think of the last time someone poked a finger into your eye!

(iii) *Mirror sign*

If you hold a mirror, or other dry, shiny surface, near the mouth, then condensation settles onto that surface from the expired air. There is no condensation of course, if the patient is dead.

(iv) *Heartbeat*

How to find the apex beat is dealt with in 'Chest Injuries'.

(v) The 'Shunting' (or 'Railroading') sign

This is a sure sign of death. It is detectable in the retina (i.e. the back of the eyeball) with the aid of an ophthalmoscope. The ophthalmoscope is an instrument which is used by doctors and opticians to detect evidence of disease in the retina. However, virtually anyone can be taught to use an ophthalmoscope well enough to detect the 'shunting' sign in the blood vessels of the retina.

The 'shunting' sign occurs at about five minutes after the circulation has stopped. It is visible up to fifteen or twenty minutes after death. After this length of time, the corneae (the 'windows' of the eyes) become opaque because the surfaces of the corneae are no longer being kept moist by secretions from the tear glands which, in life, are spread evenly over the front of the eyes by blinking actions of the eyelids.

When the circulation stops, the red blood cells, now static within the blood vessels, clump together. In the larger blood vessels, quite large clots are formed; but in the tiny blood vessels, such as those of the retina, tiny clots are formed, with serum separating one small clot from the next. These small clots can be seen in the blood vessels of the retina with the aid of an ophthalmoscope, and they look rather like a line of railway wagons in a shunting yard. Hence, the term 'shunting' or 'railroading' sign.

The appearance of this sign is delayed by any activity, which shakes the circulatory system, because any such movement agitates the red blood cells and prevents them from forming clots. Therefore, attempts at cardiopulmonary resuscitation (C.P.R.), and especially the use of the Minute-Man, will delay the appearance of the 'shunting' sign. Yet, once such activities have ceased, the observer with the ophthalmoscope can actually witness the development of the 'shunting' sign in the retinal blood vessels, and this is *a sure sign of death*.

b. Later signs of death

From the First Aider's point of view, these are: Asphyxia livida, Asphyxia pallida and Rigor mortis. I shall not discuss the effects of decomposition, because I hope that you will never have to come across the gruesome remains of anybody, weeks or months after death.

For the purposes of this description let us assume that the dead man is lying on his back.

Asphyxia pallida is a pallor of the parts of the body furthest away from the ground. In this case, that would be the face, and the front of the trunk, arms and legs. It is caused by the effect of gravity, which causes the blood in the skin to move slowly towards the ground.

Asphyxia livida occurs for the same reason. The blood which, in this case, has flowed towards the back of the head, neck, trunk, arms and legs, causes those parts of the body to have a purplish, mottled appearance, except for the parts actually in contact with the ground—i.e. the pressure points, which are actually bearing the weight of the body.

The above two processes are both part of the same gravity effect, and therefore they occur together, at the same rate. The gravity effect starts as soon as the circulation has ceased and asphyxia livida and asphyxia pallida are usually noticeable within a couple of hours.

Rigor mortis. I mentioned before that once circulation has stopped, the individual cells of the body continue to use energy until they gradually die. The muscle cells are no exception to the rule. Since the blood is no longer bringing an oxygen supply to the muscles, they have to break down their glucose supply by a very slow process. This causes the onset of a very slow contraction of the muscles, which eventually passes off when there is no further source of energy left. This process is called rigor mortis.

It is a chemical process, and chemical processes are speeded up by increasing the temperature and they are slowed down by decreasing the temperature. Thus, the speed at which rigor mortis takes place is influenced by the temperature of the environment in which the body is found. It occurs much faster in babies than in adults, because babies have a higher metabolic rate than adults.

Generally in adults in temperate climates, rigor commences at about three hours after death with stiffening of the muscles of the face, extends to the arms, hands and feet, and eventually, at about *twelve hours* after death, the whole of the body is involved in a generalised stiffness. The stiffness, or rigor, is then said to be fully established and it remains so for a further *twelve hours*. It gradually passes off during the next *twelve hours*, and from then on the body remains flaccid. The whole process of rigor is completed thirty-six hours after death.

In jungle conditions, the time taken to complete the process may be only eithteen hours, and in babies, even in temperate climates, it may be completed in nine hours.

A note of the state of rigor mortis when a body is found, and a note of the time when rigor passes off, can be *legally* important for many reasons, and can help to establish the time of death.

It should be noted that Scottish law is different from the law of England and Wales. This has always been so, and the laws relating to death are no exception to the rule. In Scotland, a dead body must be seen by a doctor as soon after death as possible. This is absolutely essential in Scottish law, but it is not necessarily so according to the law of England and Wales.

Nevertheless, as I have stated previously, it is important to be able to recognise death. This is particularly important when dealing with a number of injured people. Those who are alive and who can be restored to health, MUST be evacuated in preference to the dead. The dead must be evacuated last of all. Since there may be no doctor at the scene of the accident, the decision must be taken by the people on the spot.

4. SIMPLE FAINT (THE HIGH CLASS NAME OF THIS IS VASOVAGAL SYNOCOPE).

As I was saying, the simple faint usually occurs in a hot, humid atmosphere (typically, a crowded, poorly-ventilated room). The victim of the simple faint begins to feel weak and dizzy, starts to breathe slowly and deeply and his face becomes very pale as the blood pressure collapses and then, losing consciousness (because blood is not reaching the brain), he falls to the floor. Now, a word of caution at this point. This picture can easily be mistaken for that of a collapse following a coronary thrombosis. So, first of all allow the patient to lie flat on his back, raise the feet about one foot (30 cm) above the ground, loosen the clothing around the neck and then feel at the pulse. At first, in a simple faint, the pulse and heartbeat disappear, because the blood is pooled in the lower parts of the body and no blood is returning to the heart. Once the person is lying on the floor, the blood can flow horizontally back towards the heart, which then begins to pump blood around the circulation again. This is Nature's way of dealing with a simple faint, and it is the best way. As you feel for the radial pulse, you will feel it returning, very slowly and weakly at first, but gradually and steadily, the pulse rate and volume increase, until they are back to normal and the person regains consciousness. By raising the feet you will speed recovery by making it easier for blood to return to the heart. Until the blood returns to the heart, the person will remain unconscious, because blood and oxygen are not reaching the brain. Therefore, I will stress the following two points:

a. The person suffering from a simple faint should *ALWAYS* be allowed to lie down. You must *NEVER* prop him up against a wall or in a corner. This in turn, prolongs the brain's oxygen-lack, and *you could kill him this way!*

b. Before you dive headlong into performing external cardiac massage, *PLEASE BE SURE* that the person is not merely suffering from a simple faint!

9

The classical stages of anaesthesia

At this juncture, it is appropriate to consider the classical stages of anaesthesia. Anaesthesia is like a gentle, chemical thump on the head. The classical stages represent various levels of consciousness through which a patient would pass if anaesthesia were to be induced by the old-fashioned method of inhalation of anaesthetic vapour from a volatile liquid, such as ether or chloroform. There are four classical stages of anaesthesia. They are important in relation to endotracheal intubation and in relation to unconsciousness because they indicate the level of consciousness quite accurarely (whatever the cause of unconsciousness), be it anaesthesia, head injury or stroke.

Inhalation-induced anaesthesia takes the patient through all four of the classical stages. The original 'rag and bottle' method was to allow a few drops of anaesthetic liquid at a time to fall onto a piece of gauze which was clamped into a small metal mask held over the patient's nose and mouth. The patient inhaled the vapour from the liquid. The rate of administration of anaesthetic drops was a matter of personal judgement by the anaesthetist. This was comparable to the early aviator 'flying by the seat of his pants' in zero visibility, which, as all modern pilots know, is fraught with danger. So, just as modern aircraft have instruments which assist the pilot to fly a very accurate course, the modern anaesthetic machine has meters which measure gaseous flow rates and enable the anaesthetist to administer a very carefully controlled amount of anaesthetic.

Modern anaesthetists often induce anaesthesia by means of a basal narcotic which is a fluid and which is injected into a vein. The effect of the basal narcotic is to take the patient quickly into the third stage of anaesthesia, bypassing stages 1 and 2, just as a hefty blow to the head could throw someone into the equivalent of third stage of anaesthesia. The importance of the basal narcotic lies in bypassing stage 2 (the stage of subconscious excitement), during which stage there was an alarmingly high incidence of cardiac arrest when the 'rag and bottle' method was in common use. Flow meters, basal Narcotis and the development of low-risk anaesthetics have all helped to produce a great and most welcome decline in anaesthetic mortality. I shall now describe the classical stages of anaesthesia.

Stage 1. The stage of analgesia

Analgesia means insensitivity to pain. In this stage, the patient is still conscious, rational and orientated. His voice is guttural and his speech is slightly slurred. Respiration is regular. He is *insensitive to light pain stimulation* (e.g. pinprick), but would still appreciate heavy pain stimulation (e.g. a knuckle driven into the sternum). Analgesia is often helpful in the second stage of labour (see Pregnancy) and can be achieved by inhaling a very low dose of anaesthetic, the dose being so regulated that the woman dulls her pain but cannot render herself unconscious with it.

Stage 2. The stage of subconscious excitement

This stage has been likened to 'drunkenness'. In this stage, the respiration is stertorous (i.e. irregular, or noisy); there may even be breath-holding. The pupils are fairly dilated, as in an excited person, and the eyeballs are described as 'roving' (i.e. they move slowly or wander from side to side). There are often routine movements of the arms an legs (e.g. beating time or stamping the feet). There is often excitement, or even extreme violence. Summing these signs up, the patient can be described as *'irritable'* (see 'Head injury'— 'Level of consciousness'). The patient still responds to a heavy painful stimulus and his reflexes are still present—i.e. 'gag', swallowing, cough, vomiting, lash and corneal reflexes.

The 'gag' reflex involves the temporary blocking of the upper end of the airway by the back of the tongue. Obviously, when the tongue is so used, the person cannot speak and so is 'gagged' temporarily. The 'gag' reflex is brought into play just before swallowing or vomiting. It can be evoked by touching the rear part of the tongue or the uvula (the small, soft, pink object, which hangs from the middle of the rear edge of the soft palate.)

In Stage 1 the patient is conscious and obviously not in need of endotracheal intubation. In Stage 2 endotracheal intubation is not necessary since the 'gag', swallowing and cough reflexes are still functional. Indeed, not only is it unnecessary to intubate an unconscious person who is at this level of consciousness, but it is

POSITIVELY DANGEROUS even to attempt it, because attempted intubation at this stage is highly likely to provoke *LARYNGEAL SPASM* (i.e. spasm of the vocal cords). This effectively blocks the upper airway and causes *ASPHYXIA*, which would necessitate immediate *EMERGENCY TRACHEOTOMY* to save the patient's life. (*Even to contemplate forcing an endotracheal tube past vocal cords in spasm would be a criminally negligent act because it would cause gross and permanent damage to the vocal cords*). So, before endotracheal intubation is undertaken, there must be no doubt that the patient's level of consciousness is equivalent to either Stage 3 or Stage 4 of anaesthesia.

Stage 3. The stage of surgical anaesthesia

Obviously, this is the stage during which it is safe to carry out operations on patients. It is subdivided into Stage 3 (i) *light surgical anaesthesia* and Stage 3 (ii) *deep surgical anaesthesia*. The depth of anaesthesia is selected by the anaesthetist according to the type of operation to be performed.

The simple way to compare the two subdivisions of Stage 3 is in tabular form:

Sign	Stage 3 (i) Light	Stage 3 (ii) Deep
Respiration	Regular; deeper than normal	Regular; shallower than normal
Eyeballs	Fixed	Fixed
Pupils	Pin-point	Dilating
Reflexes (limbs, 'gag' Cough, vomiting)	Absent	Absent
Insensibility to heavy pain	Complete	Complete
Muscle relaxation	Partial	Complete
Corneal reflex	Normal	Sluggish

In Stage 3 (i) and Stage 3 (ii) it is safe to intubate the patient.

Stage 4. The stage of respiratory paralysis

This stage is often called the 'one foot in the grave' stage. In this stage, respiratory effort is absent, the pupils are widely dilated and the corneal reflex is absent. A patient can tolerate this condition for only about two minutes. If resuscitation is not undertaken very promptly, circulatory failure and death will occur. Therefore, not only is endotracheal intubation a safe procedure in Stage 4 but also it may well form an important part of resuscitation.

Endotracheal intubation is referred to again at the end of Chest injuries. There are two methods of performing intubation. The standard method is that used by anaesthetists and is called *laryngoscopic (or direct visual) intubation*, in which the anaesthetist uses an instrument called a laryngoscope. This enables him to view the vocal cords and to pass the tube under direct vision. It is undoubtedly the safer method. The second method is called *blind intubation*. In this method, a finger is passed over the back of the tongue and down towards the vocal cords in the larynx. The finger is then used as a guide for the endotracheal tube. This method has been taught to a number of ambulance personnel in the U.K. and has proved to be quite effective.

I have read one book for First Aiders in which the author describes laryngoscopic intubation. He then goes on to suggest that, having *merely read* about it, the First Aider is then capable of performing endotracheal intubation. Furthermore, he then suggests that the First Aider should acquire a laryngoscope and a set of tubes (regardless of cost) and carry them around with him, ready for instant action, without any special training other than having read about the method!

Since that author is, like myself, a member of the medical profession, I shudder to think of the potential damage to a patient's vocal cords (which could be inflicted by an untrained First Aider), quite apart from the potential legal consequences to the author! I myself would never endorse such activity by a First Aider without first ensuring that the First Aider had been properly trained, preferably by a very experienced anaesthetist.

10

Head injuries

'To explore, or not to explore the cranium?' That is the question. The decision to operate on someone who is suffering from a head injury is made by doctors in hospital. Their decision is based on the history of the injury, the findings on examination, and by observation of the progress of the injured person. This observation is carried out for twelve hours after the head injury, whether the person is conscious or not, because the first twelve hours after a head injury is the danger period, during which compression of the brain (by bleeding inside the skull) can occur. If it is more than twelve hours after the head injury, and if the patient is fully conscious, head injury observation can be discontinued.

Now the doctor can examine the patient and see the injuries for himself, but he often has to rely upon other people for the history of the injury, and neither a doctor nor a nurse in hospital can commence observation of the patient until he has reached hospital. The sooner the observation commences the better it is for patient, doctor and nurse. For example, let us suppose that a man is injured on a mountain. He is unconscious when found and because evacuation is difficult, it takes three hours to get him to hospital. If observation is begun only after he reaches hospital, then we have lost the first three recordable hours of the patient's progress. If observation begins when he is found, we have those first three hours on record and this gives us a far more complete picture of the patient's progress. The picture during those first three hours may be the factor which persuades the doctor whether to operate or not. It is especially important, too, when you bear in mind the fact that it may take an hour or two to get a rescue team up the mountain to him in the first place. *So, here is a real chance for the First Aider to shine.*

The immediate First Aid treatment of any unconscious person must be to ensure that the airway is clear and to stop haemorrhage. In fact, these are the two First Aid actions which save life more than any others. You must *NOT* however, try to stop bleeding or CSF from the nose or ears, because to do so would pre-dispose to infection. Bacteria would have an easy access to the inside of the skull and an infection inside the skull is the *last* thing a head-injury victim needs! Having taken care of the immediate First Aid, we now deal with the situation as follows:

1. History

The object here is to find out, as accurately as possible:
a. the time of the injury,
b. the duration of unconsciousness and
c. the length of retrograde amnesia (I will explain what this means later).

Every scrap of information can be vital and should be recorded, no matter how irrelevant it may seem at the time. Therefore, not only should you question the injured person if he has regained consciousness, but you should question anybody who witnessed the accident, because the injured person may not even recall the accident at all. It is quite common for him to remember events up to a few minutes before the accident, but then he remembers nothing until a point in time after the accident. In other words, he has Amnesia, (loss of memory). If we can ascertain the time of his last memory recollection *before* the accident and the time of the accident itself, then we can calculate the time of *Retrograde Amnesia*, which is the length of time between his last memory and the accident.

For example, the man with the head injury says that he remembers setting off in the morning, and he remembers the moment at which he reached the top of Scafell Pike. He remembers nothing further until he woke up and found people standing around him. Let us say that, from the man himself, and from witnesses, we ascertain that the top of Scafell Pike was reached at 10.30 a.m. and that he woke up at 11.00 a.m. The total length of amnesia is 30 minutes. However, the witnesses tell us that he fell at 10.50 a.m. Therefore the duration of Retrograde Amnesia is from 10.30 a.m. to 10.50 a.m.—20 minutes. (Retrograde means 'stepping backwards'. In this case going backwards in time from the accident.) The 10 minutes of amnesia *following* the injury (going foward in time from the accident) is known as anterograde amnesia.

Before we proceed any further. I owe you an explanation and a word of caution. Our brains perform many functions, one of which is memory-storage. Facts and events can be stored in the brain, just as they can in a computer. However, just as it takes time to programme a computer, so it takes a little time to store facts in the brain. The whole purpose of storing facts in our brains is to enable us to recall those facts for use at a later date. The most important facts are stored indefinitely (everyone knows his own date of birth), but the relatively unimportant facts are stored for only a very short time (e.g. most of us could not recall what we ate for lunch on 19th April, 1973, unless of course, it was a day to remember, such as friend's wedding day!) A blow to the head can interfere with the memory storage process. This explains why the victim of a head injury cannot recall events for a certain length of time. He cannot recall events because his brain has *been unable to store them*. That is the explanation. The importance of assessing the length of retrograde amnesia as accurately as possible is that *the length of retrograde amnesia is directly proportional to the severity of the head injury*.

Now, let me caution you about the wily ways of *Anterograde Amnesia*. Let us take the same example but with a slight modification. The man remembers reaching the top of Scafell Pike at 10.30 a.m. and the witnesses confirm this. The witnesses maintain that he fell at 10.50 a.m. and that he woke up at 11.00 a.m. Furthermore the witnesses say that he was able to get up, he appeared perfectly normal, could speak and answer questions rationally, and he even walked back to base. Our man on the other hand, states quite categorically that he remembers nothing after reaching the top of Scafell Pike until they were arriving back at the base, which was at 11.30 a.m. What a peculiar conflict of stories! Is our man lying, or did everybody else mistake the time? In fact, nobody is mistaken. It is the same problem of inability to store memories in the injured brain. *The man's memory-storage function did not recover until 11.30 a.m.*, although he was conscious and rational from 11.00 a.m. In this case, therefore, we have anterograde amnesia of 40 minutes (i.e. from 10.50 a.m., when he was injured to 11.30 a.m.) This includes 10 minutes of unconsciousness. We also have the same 20 minutes of retrograde amnesia.

Anterograde amnesia is not very important from a First Aider's point of view, and you should not waste time trying to puzzle it out. I merely wanted to warn you that it can have puzzling effects. Your main aim, in taking the history is to assess as accurately as possible the three things I mentioned initially—i.e. the time of injury, the duration of unconsciousness and the length of retrograde amnesia. Once you have assessed these three things, write them down, concisely and *LEGIBLY*, e.g.:

'Time of injury = 10.50 a.m. Witnesses confirm this.'

'Unconsciousness = 10 minutes. Witnesses confirm this (woke up at 11.00 a.m.)'

'Retrograde amnesia = 20 minutes—Patient remembers top of Scafell Pike at 10.30 a.m.'

In these three lines you have covered the essential points of the history.

If the patient has not recovered consciousness, you cannot assess the length of retrograde amnesia, because you cannot question him. You would then write.

Time of injury = 10.50 a.m.—witnesses confirm this.

Patient still unconscious at . . . (time you reach him).

2. Examination

Having safeguarded the airway and arrested haemorrhage, approach the patient as described in Part II. Feel at the pulse and look at the face, whether he is conscious or not. If the signs of shock are present—pallor, cold, clammy skin and a rapid, thready pulse—then be on the look-out for other injuries, apart from the head injury, because shock is *not* usually a feature of head injury. When we use the word 'Shock' on its own, we are referring to the general condition of the patient which is produced by gross blood loss, stove-in chest injury, or a penetrating wound of the abdomen. Gross blood loss would be the result of external haemorrhage, or of bleeding internally into the abdomen or thorax (chest), or of blood loss from fractures. So, if you do find the signs of shock in someone with a head injury, *beware!* A certain amount of pallor of the face may be seen in someone who has just recovered from being unconscious, but the skin is not cold and clammy and there is no rapid, thready pulse. This pallor is due to concussion. *Concussion* simply means brain injury and the diagnosis of concussion can be made when a person, who has had a blow to the head, has retrograde amnesia. He usually has a headache too!

Let us proceed with the examination. Having felt at the pulse and looked at the face, we then look for bleeding and/or CSF from the nose and ears, and we feel for lacerations, depressions, haematomas and oedema. Lacerations are easily felt, so is the blood from them. Depressions in the skull are surprisingly difficult to feel. A *haematoma* is a collection of blood in soft tissues. It can occur anywhere, but in this context, a haematoma would lie between the skull and scalp. On pressing upon it with your fingers (as if you were playing a piano) it would feel crinkly, rather like a piece of soggy tissue paper. *Oedema* is a soft-tissue swelling caused by an increase of fluid amongst the cells in the soft tissue. The fluid does not form a pool, but is interspersed among the cells. If you come across this swelling and you press your finger into it for about five seconds, you will find that the pressure of your finger has left an indentation, or a 'pit mark'. This pitting is typical of oedema. If it is found on the scalp, it is virtually always indicative of a skull fracture and the fracture is usually directly underneath the oedema. In other words, *oedema of the scalp is virtually diagnostic of a skull fracture and it marks the fracture site*. Observe the pupils at this stage.

The rest of the examination should be carried out as described in Part II. Make a list of all injuries found, and indicate with drawings where any lacerations, haematomas or oedema of the scalp are found. (See also The search for injuries in the unconscious patient, p. 206).

3. Observation

I have already explained the reason for this. For the sake of completeness, the nurses in hospital take the patient's blood pressure and temperature each time they observe the patient. Unfortunately it is not practical for a mountain rescue team to take the blood pressure and temperature every fifteen to thirty minutes during the evacuation of the patient, because he is firmly strapped down to a stretcher. If you wish, you may take the blood pressure and temperature when you examine the patient initially. The periodic observation which you will be able to carry out, during evacuation of the patient, will be of the other five factors, which are observed when the patient is under observation in hospital. These are: (i) Pulse, (ii) Pupils, (iii) Respiration, (iv) Level of consciousness and (v) Level of response.

(i) *The pulse*

Even though the patient may be strapped firmly to a stretcher, you can arrange it so that you are able to assess the patient's radial or carotid pulse. Remember, you want to record the rate, rhythm and volume of the pulse; e.g. '60/min regular, normal', or it may be '90/min irregular, feeble'. Accepted abbreviations are 'reg' for regular and 'irreg' irregular.

(ii) Pupils

These should be observed for the following:

a. Size—whether constricted, normal or dilated (e.g. Right dilated; Left normal).

b. Reaction to light—brisk, normal, sluggish or absent. You should always check for the Consensual light reflex, too. To do this, shine a light into one eye and shield the other eye from the torchlight. The pupil of the eye into which the light is shone normally constricts. So, too, does the pupil of the other eye, even though the light is not shining into it. The second pupil is, in fact, constricting in sympathy with the first pupil. This is the consensual light reflex. So, your record might be: 'Reaction normal; Right and Left, consensual reflex normal'. *Please do not* write R for right and L for left. The *written* capitals R and L can be mistaken for each other. You may find this hard to believe, but it is true.

(iii) Respiration

We want to know the rate and type of respiration. The rate of respiration can be counted. The types are: normal, shallow, deep, stertorous (noisy) or Cheyne-Stokes. There could also be deep, sighing respiration as in air hunger. Your record of respiration, for example, might be, '23/min shallow'. In Cheyne-Stokes respiration which is crescendo breathing with periods of apnoea (no breathing) the rate of respiration varies, of course. Therefore, you simply record 'Cheyne-Stokes'.

(iv) Level of consciousness

Various diagrammatic methods of representing the level of consciousness have been devised, but they are not satisfactory. Let us take, for example, the method of shading in part of a square. One observer's *impression* of the state of consciousness of a patient may be to shade in a quarter of the square, whilst another observer's impression of the same patient's state of consciousness may be to fill in half a square. It is far better, therefore, to use a system of *words*, which we all understand. These words are:

a. Conscious.

b. Orientated (knows where he is and what is happening).

c. Disorientated (does not know where he is. He is confused).

   d. Irritable   Self explanatory.
   e. Drowsy
   f. Rouseable (goes to sleep but can be awakened).
   g. Unrouseable (asleep and cannot be awakened).

If you use these words, your record will be understood by hospital staff.

(v) *Level of response*

Just as with level of consciousness, a system of words is by far the best means of recording the level of response. We record as follows:
Responds to:
   a. Normal voice
   b. Shouting
   c. Tickling
   d. Turning over
   e. Pressure
   f. Pain (e.g. nipping the skin)
   g. Severe pain (e.g. drive a knuckle firmly into the middle of your own breast bone. You will find it quite painful)
   h. Unresponsive (i.e. does not respond to any of the above).

Again, by using this system of words, your record will be understood by hospital staff. That is very important for the continuity of the treatment of the patient, once he has reached hospital.

In conclusion, I would stress the following points:

(i) Your history, examination and observation should follow the above scheme.

(ii) Your records should be legible. Other people have to read them!

(iii) Your observations should be carried out every fifteen minutes, if possible. Every thirty minutes is acceptable, especially if evacuation is long and difficult.

(iv) Finally, I would suggest that you contact the hospital in your area, so that you may see how the hospital head injury record sheet is printed. You can then arrange it so that the format of your head injury record corresponds to that of the hospital. This will eliminate another possible source of confusion. Some hospitals use charts which combine the records of head injury and multiple injuries, and this type of chart is known as a Major Accident Record.

I have already explained what is meant by concussion, but before I leave the subject of head injuries, I would like to clarify what is meant by *Compression*. A depressed fracture of the skull may exert

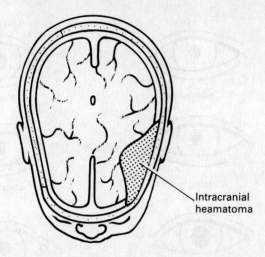

Fig. 28 Intracranial haematoma causing brain compression.

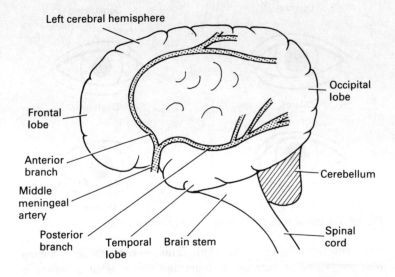

Fig. 29 Rupture of the middle meningeal artery is the usual cause of brain compression.

a small amount of pressure on the brain, but this pressure does *not* continue to increase. However, when there is bleeding inside the skull, the blood cannot escape and it cannot expand the rigid skull vault. Therefore, the increasing pool of blood has no alternative but

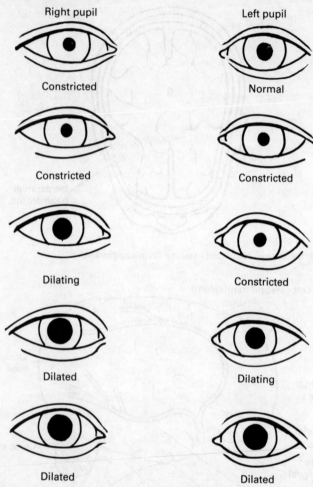

Right pupil

Left pupil

Constricted

Normal

Constricted

Constricted

Dilating

Constricted

Dilated

Dilating

Dilated

Dilated

Fig. 30 The typical sequence of pupil changes in compression.

to extend inwards, inside the skull. This, in turn, causes a *continuous, progressive pressure on the brain* and this is what is meant by compression.

Let us consider the classical example of compression. This occurs as a rupture of the Middle Meningeal Artery, which is a small artery inside the skull, running along the inner surface of the temporal bone. The typical story is that the injured person received a blow to the temple. He may or may not have been unconscious. Either way, he seemed to have recovered well enough. Later, perhaps after a few hours, he complained of a headache, vomited and became

drowsy. He would then gradually pass into unrouseable unconsciousness and unresponsiveness, and we would also see the pupils
change. Depending upon whether the bleeding is occurring inside
the right side or the left side of the skull, one side of the brain is
compressed first, usually the side of the brain on the same side as
the bleeding. (Occasionally, the opposite side of the brain is affected first). A typical sequence of pupil changes would be as follows:

Stage 1. Left pupil constricts (Right pupil still normal)
     2. Right pupil constricts (Both now constricted)
     3. Left pupil dilates (Right pupil still constricted)
     4. Right pupil dilates (Both dilated).

In about 85 per cent of cases, the pupil on the same side as the
bleeding constricts first. In about 15 per cent of cases, the opposite
pupil constricts first. *The importance of the first aider's function is to
recognise the typical sequence of pupil changes which denote compression.*
(Localisation of the site of compression is the function of the
neurosurgeon.)

When Stage 4 is reached, neither pupil will react to light, and
the corneal reflex will soon disappear. The blood pressure, pulse
rate and volume, and respiratory rate and volume will probably
have all increased by this time, and all of them will soon fall fairly
quickly to nothing. The patient may exhibit Cheyne-Stokes respiration before he dies. This is the classical picture of Compression.
It is stressed because if the skull is explored in time, the bleeding
can be stopped, the blood clot evacuated, and the patient can be
restored dramatically to a normal state of physical and mental health.

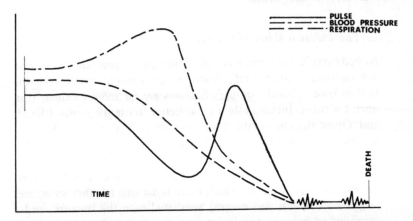

Fig. 31 Typical progressive changes in pulse rate, blood pressure, and respiratory
rate during the late stages of the brain compression.

11

Injuries to bones and joints

The fractures which can occur in the various bones of the body, and how to deal with those fractures, are dealt with quite adequately in the First Aid Manuals. I will not waste your time by repeating a whole list of fractures. I will remind you of the 'give-away' signs and the 'head-to-toe' method of examination, which I described when discussing the search for injuries. I will remind you, also, that some fractures may be painless for a few hours after injury, because of the adrenaline response, that the patient may have referred pain, and that the pain of one fracture may mask the pain from another. These facts serve to emphasise the importance of *feeling* for tenderness and/or crepitus. The patient should be examined from head to toe. Any points of tenderness should be noted as you go along. When you have been over the patient from head to toe, you can then examine the tender places in more detail. I shall now deal with the cardinal signs of fracture, a few general points about joint injuries and the estimation of blood loss from fractures, in that order.

1. The cardinal signs of fracture

Nobody has X-ray eyes, and unless we come across somebody who has an open ('compound') fracture, we cannot actually see the broken bone. Closed ('simple') fractures are far more common than open fractures. Incidentally it is far better to use the terms 'Closed' and 'Open' than to use the terms 'Simple' or 'Compound'. The reason for this is that the word 'Simple', in everyday language, is the opposite of 'Complicated', and therefore, when talking of fractures, the terms 'Compound' and 'Complicated' can be confused. A *complicated* fracture is one in which there is damage to other structures (e.g. blood vessels and nerves) associated with the fracture, and a complicated fracture may be open or closed. So, please try to avoid the use of the words 'Simple' and 'Compound'.

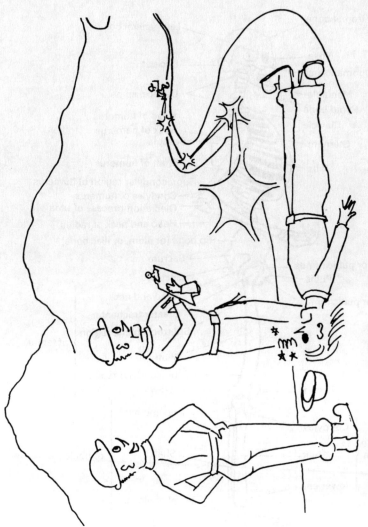

Fig. 32 Adrenaline response positive, Joe.

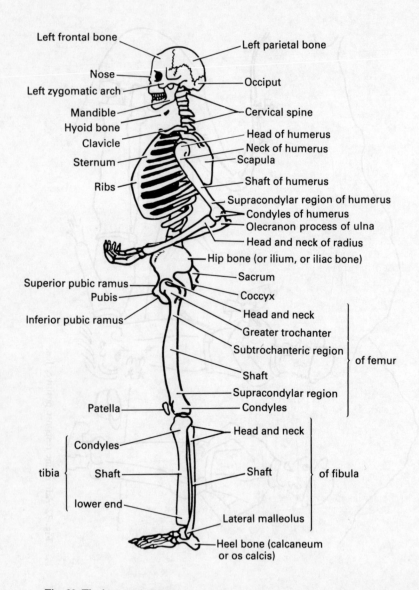

Fig. 33 The human skeleton.

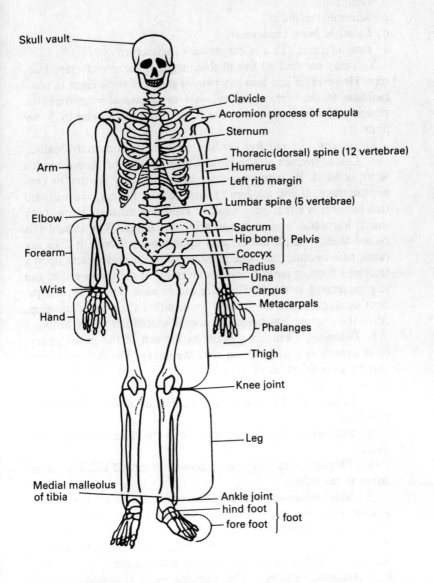

Skull vault

Clavicle
Acromion process of scapula
Sternum
Thoracic (dorsal) spine (12 vertebrae)
Humerus
Left rib margin
Lumbar spine (5 vertebrae)

Arm

Elbow

Forearm

Wrist

Hand

Sacrum
Hip bone } Pelvis
Coccyx
Radius
Ulna
Carpus
Metacarpals
Phalanges

Thigh

Knee joint

Leg

Medial malleolus
of tibia

Ankle joint
hind foot } foot
fore foot

Since the First Aider cannot take X-ray films, he has to rely on the five cardinal signs of fracture, which are:

a. Loss of function.

b. Deformity.

c. Abnormal mobility.

d. *Localised* bony tenderness.

e. *Bony* crepitus (This is diagnostic of a fracture).

You may not find all five of these signs at the site of every fracture. However, if you find any two, or more, of these signs in combination at the site of injury, you can reasonably assume the presence of a fracture at that site, until proved otherwise by X-ray films.

Let us consider our five cardinal signs of fracture individually.

a. Loss of function.   The patient may say that he cannot use his wrist, or hand. By your own observation, you may see that he cannot use them. If you ask him to squeeze your fingers, you will find that his grip is either very weak or even non-existent. He will say that it hurts him to even try to grip your finger. Why should this be so? Well, when a muscle acts upon a normal bone it does not cause pain because the bone is intact. When a muscle acts upon a fractured bone, it tends to cause movement at the fracture site, and any movement at the fracture site causes pain. Therefore, the patient declines to use the injured limb, rather than suffer the pain. Also, the fracture has upset the normal mechanics of the limb.

b. Deformity.   This may occur as a result of the initial injury, or as a result of muscle spasm after the injury. The deformity itself may be a combination of any of the four different types of deformity, which are:

(i) Angulation—i.e. one fragment forms an abnormal angle with the other.

(ii) Rotation—i.e. one fragment may twist in relation to the other.

(iii) Displacement—i.e. one fragment is moved sideways in relation to the other.

(iv) Shortening—i.e. the fragments override each other, causing a shortening of (say) one femur compared with the other. The shortening is actually caused by spasm of the thigh muscles. This muscle spasm occurs reflexly after injury, and it tends to reduce movement (and therefore pain) at the fracture site.

c. Abnormal mobility.   This explains itself. If movement occurs where it should not, e.g. in the middle of the tibia and fibula—this is abnormal mobility.

d. Localised bony tenderness. Localised is the key word here. Generalised bony tenderness may occur if a bone is bruised. Tenderness localised to one particular point of the bone should make you suspicious of a fracture. It is worth noting, too, that where a bone lies just under the skin (e.g. skull, tibia, ulna and clavicle) there may be *oedema* at the fracture site. (Oedema was referred to in 'Head Injuries').

e. Bony crepitus. This is a rather unpleasant crunching sound, caused by any movement which results in the grating together of the fragments of the broken bone. Apart from being an unpleasant sound, bony crepitus causes the patient considerable pain. For this reason you should never search for it deliberately. If you do hear it, or feel it, then it is diagnostic of a fracture. I emphasise the term 'bony crepitus' because there is also soft-tissue crepitus, which is quite different and which will be referred to when we consider 'Chest Injuries'.

These then, are the five cardinal signs of fracture, and you should remember them, because (apart from the 'give-away' signs) they are the only guides which the First Aider can rely on when trying to rule out fracture, or to make a diagnosis of fracture.

Two other signs, which can occur with fractures, but which are not cardinal signs, are:

(i) *Oedema*, which has been referred to already under 'Localised bony tenderness', and

(ii) *Ecchymosis*. In appearance, this is like bruising. In fact, it is blood from a fracture site which has migrated under the effect of gravity over a period of two or three days to another part of the body—e.g. from the neck of the humerus to the elbow. Therefore, it differs from bruising in that (a) it is not tender, whereas bruising is tender, and (b) it is found remote from the site of injury, whereas bruising occurs at the site of injury.

2. Joint injuries

Swellings in joints caused by injury cannot be diagnosed accurately without X-ray films. Therefore, it would be grossly unfair to expect a First Aider to make an accurate diagnosis of a swollen joint. So, if a joint is swollen, simply splint it and take the patient to hospital. Before going further, I will caution you *against* trying to manipulate a dislocation, or fracture-dislocation. The ability to manipulate successfully and *safely* depends on two things. Firstly, the manipulator must have an inborn knack for manipulation and this is composed of three things:

a. the ability to use *controlled* strength to a very fine degree;
b. a *very* sensitive touch;
c. the ability to hold a mental picture of what is happening to a joint, as he manipulates it.

Secondly, the manipulator must have been through a course of *training*. So, the general rule for First Aiders is NOT to manipulate joints. However, having said that, I think you should be aware of the injuries which can occur to joints, because it will make you more aware of the need for X-ray films before a diagnosis can be made. I will list the injuries first, and then discuss them. The injuries are:

(i) Sprain.
(ii) Contusion (internal bruising).
(iii) Internal derangement.
(iv) Fracture into a joint.
(v) Dislocation.
(vi) Fracture-dislocation.
(vii) Pulled elbow (in children).

After many joint injuries, a fluid swelling occurs in the joint. The joint swells up and if you squeeze *gently* your fingers can feel the fluid fluctuate under their pressure. This fluid swelling is called an *Effusion*, and an effusion, after injury, may be composed of:

a. synovial fluid,
b. blood, or
c. a mixture of both.

The history can give us a good idea of what kind of effusion it is. If the patient says that the joint had swollen up within fifteen to twenty minutes, then it is 'odds-on' that the effusion is blood. If the swelling occurred, say, up to an hour after the injury, the effusion is probably a mixture of blood and synovial fluid. If it took longer than an hour for the swelling to develop, then that effusion is highly likely to be composed of synovial fluid alone. These effusions are seen quite frequently in the knee, ankle, elbow, wrist and finger joints. Now, let us discuss the injuries.

(i) A sprain

This is an injury which causes stretching of the capsule and the synovial membrane of a joint. The synovial membrane responds to the injury by pouring out excessive synovial fluid, to form an effusion. If there is a small tear in the synovial membrane, the fluid will contain some blood. (*N.B.* the word *Strain* should not be used to describe a joint injury. A strain is a stretching injury of a tendon or muscle.)

(ii) A contusion

This is a form of internal bruising, caused by a jolting injury to the joint. The jolting blow causes temporary damage to the articular cartilage which covers each bone end. As a result of this, the articular cartilages lose their ability to move against each other smoothly, and any attempted movement causes pain. In order to try to compensate for this, the synovial membrane pours out much more of the lubricating synovial fluid than usual, the object being that the fluid should separate the articular cartilages, restore smooth movement and ease pain. So much fluid is needed to do this, however, that the effusion bulges the joint capsule, and this in itself causes aching. Overall, the general effect of the effusion is a reduction of pain caused by the contusion. Contusion of the elbow and knee are quite common.

(iii) A fracture into a joint

This causes an effusion of blood into that joint, because the fracture-line has breached the articular cartilage, and the way is clear for blood to flow from the fracture-site into the joint. The joints commonly involved in this kind of injury are the elbow, the knee and the ankle. The swelling of the joint occurs within fifteen to twenty minutes after the injury. The lesson to be learned here is that, *if you have reason to believe that an effusion has been caused by bleeding into a joint, then it is reasonable to suspect a fracture involving that joint, until you are proved wrong by X-rays.*

(iv) Internal derangements

I have put this in for the sake of completeness. These internal derangements are outside the First Aider's diagnostic scope but you should be aware of them. The knee is the prize example. The knee joint contains four structures, which are as follows:

(a) *The medial meniscus and* (b) *the lateral meniscus.* These menisci are commonly known as cartilages. The medial one lies on the medial side of the joint, (nearer the midline of the body). The lateral one lies on the lateral side of the joint, away from the midline of the body. They are both roughly 'new moon' shaped and their function is to facilitate rotational movements of the knee joint.

(c) *The anterior cruciate ligament.* The function of this ligament is to prevent the femur from sliding too far backwards on the upper surface of the tibia.

(d) *The posterior cruciate ligament* prevents the femur from sliding too far forwards on the upper surface of the tibia. These cruciate ligaments are so called because they cross over each other, within the joint. (Actually, from a strictly anatomical point of view, they are outside the knee joint proper, but that need not worry the First Aider. These ligaments *function* as an integral part of the knee joint). If any undue strain is placed upon the knee, then any of the four structures I have just mentioned can be damaged, whether there is any bony damage or not.

The medial and lateral collateral ligaments lie outside the knee joint, but they add stability and prevent the knee from bending in the wrong direction (see *Examination of the Knee*, in Part II).

The medial collateral ligament lies outside the medial (inner) aspect of the knee joint. It prevents the medial side of the joint from opening up, when a strain is applied to the fully-extended knee from the lateral (outer) aspect—i.e. it prevents the knee from bending so that the leg angles laterally (outwards). If the leg can be made to angle this way, then the medial collateral ligament has been torn.

The lateral collateral ligament functions similarly, by preserving the stability of the lateral side of the knee joint.

(v) Dislocation

This is defined as 'complete loss of apposition of the articular surfaces of a joint' (i.e. complete loss of the normal relationship of one joint surface to another). You may have heard of the word '*Subluxation*'. This is a partial dislocation (i.e. incomplete loss of the normal relationship of joint surfaces).

Dislocation of the shoulder is quite common. It can be recognised by the following signs:

a. Flattened deltoid muscle (one of the 'give-away' signs described in Part II.)

b. Inability to touch the tip of the uninjured shoulder with the fingers of the hand of the same side as the injured shoulder (e.g.

if the right shoulder is dislocated, the patient cannot touch the tip of his left shoulder with his right fingers).

Dislocation of the elbow is fairly common, and is easy to diagnose if you know the bony landmarks around the elbow. In this condition, the upper end of the ulna is pushed backwards with respect to the lower end of the humerus, and (unless the radius is fractured) the upper end of the radius is pushed upwards, with respect to the lower end of the humerus. The overall effect of dislocation of the elbow is shortening of the forearm. Shortening of the forearm can also be caused by fractures of the radius and ulna. Therefore, if you find a dislocation of the head of the radius (upper end) *without* dislocation of the upper end of the ulna (the olecranon process), you *must* search for a fracture of the shaft of the ulna, which would allow shortening of the forearm and, hence, dislocation of the head of the radius. Having warned you of this pitfall, I must confess that I have seen a few dislocations of the head of the radius without fracture of the ulna. In those cases, the only rational explanation can be that there was a subluxation of the inferior radio-ulnar joint (i.e. a partial dislocation of the joint between the lower ends of the radius and ulna, just above the wrist joint).

The bony landmarks of the elbow. Let us now indulge in a little practical amusement by finding these landmarks. If you cannot remember the names of these landmarks, it does not matter. The important thing is that you should be able to find them. You should always examine the patient's left elbow with your right hand, and his right elbow with your left hand. This is easy to remember because you cannot possibly touch your right elbow with your right hand, nor can you touch your left elbow with your left hand. Therefore, you can practise on your own elbows correctly. Apart from examining for a full range of movements at the elbow joint, we want to be able to find three things, *viz*:

a. the normal bony triangle of the elbow. If this is lost, then there is a dislocation or a fracture-dislocation of the elbow.

b. the normal position of the head of the radius. This normally rotates smoothly, when the forearm is pronated and supinated. If the head of the radius is tender, or if there is crepitus on pronation and supination, suspect a fracture of the head of the radius. If it is out of its normal position then it is dislocated.

c. any effusion which may be present.

a. *To find the bony triangle in your own left elbow*, first place your left elbow at a right angle, with the palm facing upwards. Now, place the palm of your right hand under the back of your left fore-arm, with the fingers pointing towards the left elbow. Slide your right hand towards the left elbow and when you reach the elbow, do the following three things:

(1) With your right *Index* finger, find the 'point' of the elbow. This is the tip of the olecranon process of the ulna. Keep your right index finger on this point.

(2) With your right *middle* finger, search about on the medial side of the elbow (the side nearer to the body) and at about one or one-and-a-half inches away from the tip of the olecranon, you will find another bony point. This is the medial epicondyle of the humerus. Keep your middle finger on it.

(3) With your right *thumb*, search on the lateral (outer) side of the elbow and you will find another bony point, again about one or one-and-a-half inches away from the tip of the olecranon. This is the lateral epicondyle of the humerus. Keep your thumb on it.

With your thumb, index and middle fingers covering their respective bony landmarks, you will see that they form a triangle, because *when the elbow is flexed to a right angle*, they all lie in the same plane. If the elbow is fully extended, the triangle disappears, and all the points come to lie in a straight line. Try it! This should serve to remind you that the elbow must be at a right angle, if you are to find the bony triangle.

If you are examining someone else's left elbow, then hold his left hand in yours, as if shaking hands. Your left hand can then be used to hold his elbow at a right angle and your right hand is free to examine the elbow.

b. *To find the head of your own left radius*, simply find the lateral epicondyle of the humerus (the one you found with your right thumb, before) and place the tip of your right middle finger onto it, with your right fingers pointing towards your left shoulder. If you now place the tip of your right index finger next to the tip of the middle finger, you should feel the head of the radius. When you rotate your left forearm (i.e. pronate and supinate it) you will feel the head of the radius rotate beneath the tip of your right index finger. When practising this on someone else, you should use your left hand to rotate his left forearm by the 'hand shaking' method, and your right hand to rotate his right forearm.

c. *Effusions*, when present, produce a bulging of the capsule of the elbow joint. This bulging can be felt either between the tip of the olecranon and the medial epicondyle, or between the tip of the olecranon and the lateral epicondyle, when the elbow is held at a right angle.

With a little practice you should be able to find the normal bony triangle, the head of the radius and any effusion present in about ten seconds flat, if not less. You have no excuse for not practising how to find the bony landmarks. You have two hands and two elbows, and where you go, they go!

Dislocation of the patella is not uncommon and is often *recurrent* (i.e. the patient will tell you that it has happened previously). The patella slips laterally (i.e. towards the outer side of the knee, away from the midline of the body). Quite often, it slips back into its normal position when the knee is straightened. If it does, all well and good—just apply a bandage for support. If it does not slip back into position spontaneously you must *not* try to force it back.

(*vi*) Fracture-dislocation

This is dislocation complicated by a fracture, or fractures. Good examples of fracture-dislocation occur in the shoulder, elbow and hip. Sir Percival Pott who was a surgeon in London in the eighteenth century, described a fracture-dislocation of the ankle joint. This came to be known as 'Pott's Fracture'. Unfortunately, the term 'Pott's Fracture' has been used far too loosely for far too long. Nowadays, people often use the term quite wrongly, to describe any type of fracture or fracture-subluxation of the ankle joint (i.e. a fracture of the ankle joint with incomplete dislocation). Therefore, the term 'Pott's Fracture' is best avoided unless you are absolutely sure that the ankle is

a. *fractured* and
b. *dislocated*.

Dislocation and fracture-dislocation of the hip can both be caused by the same kinds of accidents (car crashes, coal-mining and mountaineering accidents). In either case, the hip may be flexed, adducted and internally rotated (as described in Part II). X-ray films are needed to differentiate dislocation from fracture-dislocation of the hip. This is an important point. The mechanism of injury involved in the production of dislocation of the hip is quite different from the mechanism of injury by which a fracture-dislocation occurs. Because of these differences in mechanism of injury, the methods of manipulation of these two injuries are quite different. So, without X-ray films, we do not know which method of manipulation to use. In any case, the manipulation of a hip joint can be very difficult. THEREFORE, ON NO ACCOUNT MUST YOU EVER TRY TO MANIPULATE A HIP JOINT!

The signs of fracture-dislocation of the shoulder and the elbow are the same as for dislocation. The fractures are usually noticed on X-ray films. Fracture-subluxation of the ankle joint is fairly common, whilst fracture-dislocation (the true Pott's Fracture) is very rare indeed. Dislocations of the joints of the fingers and thumbs are fairly common, and the deformity is usually quite obvious. Dislocation of the knee joint (as opposed to dislocation of the patella) is very rare.

(vii) Pulled elbow

This is a condition which occurs in young children. It is a very painful injury and, if not treated early, the child will remain in pain and be unable to use the affected limb for a few days. The injury is caused by a jerking force along the fully-extended upper limb, and this causes the radius to slide away from the humerus. As it slides away from the humerus, the head of the radius becomes wedged into the annular ligament. Now, this annular ligament is a circular, tough ligament. It is attached to the upper end of the ulna, and normally it encircles the neck of the radius (the part just below the head of the radius). Its *normal* function is to prevent the upper end of the radius from splaying away from the upper end of the ulna, whilst at the same time allowing the radius to rotate freely. In the case of a 'pulled elbow', the function of the annular ligament is abnormal, because the head of the radius is wedged firmly into it. Thereby, free rotation of the radius has been lost, and any attempt to rotate the radius causes severe pain.

The history is usually obtained from the parents. They may tell you that the child was holding a rail when he fell, still holding the rail. Very commonly, the mother will tell you that they were walking along the pavement, hand in hand, when the child slipped off the edge of the kerb, and she pulled him up by the hand to prevent him from falling into the road. In either case, the mechanism of injury is a jerking force acting along the fully-extended upper limb and the result is the same. The child lets the injured limb hang limply to his side and he will not even *attempt* to use it, no matter how you coax him. If you ask his mother to take a firm grip on his *un*injured arm and then offer him a chocolate or a toy, he will struggle to try to free his uninjured arm, rather than try to use the injured one. If he had a greenstick fracture of the clavicle, or upper end of humerus, or lower end of radius, he would *at least try* to use the injured limb. The child himself, is usually crying, or may cry intermittently, and he usually complains of pain at the elbow. Sometimes however, he complains of pain at the wrist. This is because the sliding movement of the radius has not only wedged the head of the radius into the annular ligament, but it has also caused a subluxation of the inferior radio-ulnar joint (i.e. the joint between the lower ends of the radius and ulna, just above the wrist joint).

The diagnosis of 'pulled elbow' is made from the history, which is typical, and from the finding of a limp, loosely-hanging upper limb, which the child refuses to use. The treatment is by manipulation, which must NEVER be performed before an X-ray has been taken to rule out the possibility of a fracture.

3. Estimation of potential blood loss from fractures

In Part I, I stated that broken bones bleed. I pointed out that the blood which oozes out of a broken bone into the tissues is lost from the circulation, just as surely as if it had poured onto the ground. Loss of blood from the circulation affects the general condition of the patient and the greater the blood loss, the greater its effect on the general condition. As this blood loss takes place over a few hours, it may take a few hours for the patient's general condition to deteriorate, but deteriorate it will, especially in a patient with multiple fractures. Just now rapidly we can expect a patient's general condition to deteriorate after injury depends on an estimation of *the total potential blood loss*. This estimation helps us to determine our order of priority of evacuation, when dealing with mass casualties. The general condition of the patient with the greatest *potential* blood loss can be expected to deteriorate faster than the general condition of the other injured people, and this gives him priority of evacuation over them. The following list is a good guide to the estimation of the total blood loss of an injured person:

Estimation of potential Blood Loss

Fracture of:

Clavicle	$\frac{1}{4}$ pint
Humerus (any part)	$\frac{1}{2}$–1 pint
Forearm bones (one or both) ...	$\frac{1}{2}$–1 pint
Hand & Wrist	usually negligible
Spinal bones	usually negligible

Pelvis	2–4 pints
Grossly fractured, unstable pelvis	up to 8 pints
Femur (any part)	2–3 pints
Tibia (any part)	1–2 pints
Fibula	$\frac{1}{4}$ pint
Foot (any part)	$\frac{1}{4}$ pint
Ankle	$\frac{1}{4}$–$\frac{1}{2}$ pint

I must emphasise that the above list is a *guide*. You may have seen similar lists, and you may have noted one or two discrepancies between those lists and this one, but please remember that these are estimates and not exact measurements. In any case the discrepancies between this list and any other should not be very great. So, please do not argue about which list is right and which is wrong. There is no exact right and wrong in an estimate of any kind, since, by definition, an estimate is a reasonably accurate assessment of something.

In practice, I use this list in the following way. I list the fractures found, add up the *potential minimum* and the *potential maximum* blood loss from them, and then take a figure half-way between the two totals. This figure I accept as the total potential blood loss of that person. This figure is also the number of pints of blood I would request for transfusion into that person. For example, if the minimum estimate is six pints and the maximum is ten pints, the figure half-way between these two is eight pints. So, I would accept eight pints as his potential blood loss and I would request eight pints of blood for transfusion into him. His response to the blood transfusion will determine whether or not he needs any more blood after the first eight pints.

Before I leave the subject of blood loss estimation, I should point out that blood loss within the abdomen or chest may have to be taken into account, too. I would also remind you of Air Hunger (see *Facial Appearance* Part II) and of the fact that the spleen carries a reserve supply of red blood cells which can be released into the circulation in an emergency (see Part I).

People with multiple fractures should be monitored prior to evacuation to hospital. The pulse, blood pressure and respiration should be *recorded*, preferably every fifteen minutes, up to the time of evacuation of that person. I shall elaborate on this, when I deal with 'Mass Casualties'.

Relief of pain in fractures and dislocations is rather a moot point at present. Many First Aiders have asked me about this, either because they are worried about having to give an injection, or about what they would have to inject. There could also be legal problems in allowing a First Aider to carry any potential drug of addiction, such as morphine or pethidine. Quite frankly, my own view is that First Aiders do not need to give injections, nor do they need to carry around dangerous drugs. There is a drug on the market now, which is called pentazocine hydrochloride (trade name 'Fortral') and this drug can be obtained in the form of suppositories. These are easily inserted into the rectum, well absorbed from the rectum and there is no problem about sterility, as there is with injections. Furthermore, pentazocine hydrochloride is not classed as a dangerous drug, and it is as strong a pain-killer as morphine. The only drawback is that it has a morphine-like action on the pupils (it causes the pupils to constrict). Therefore it must *not* be given to anyone who has sustained a head injury. Pentazocine hydrochloride is available as suppositories, 50 mg each, and also as injections, 30 mg and 60 mg per ampoule.

In all fairness to those who prefer to use the more traditional pain-killers, I should make mention of morphine, pethidine and papaveretum (Trade name, 'Omnopon'). All three of these are derived from opium. Opium is not one chemical compound, but a mixture of chemical compounds. Morphine and pethidine are pure chemical compounds derived from opium. They are strong pain-killers, but have a tendency to cause vomiting. However, they do have a sedative effect, not possessed by pentazocine hydrochloride. Papaveretum is a mixture of compounds derived from opium. It is as good a pain-killer as morphine and pethidine, has a better sedative effect and does not cause vomiting to the same extent. Morphine, pethidine and papaveretum tend to depress blood pressure, whereas pentazocine hydrochloride tends to cause a slight increase in blood pressure. Morphine is available in ampoules of 10 mg, 20 mg and 30 mg; Pethidine in ampoules of 50 mg and 100 mg, and papaveretum in ampoules of 10 mg and 20 mg. Legally, only doctors and certain members of the nursing profession are allowed to be in possession of drugs derived from opium, apart from pharmacists who are allowed to stock these drugs, and certain specialised First Aiders.

I have mentioned but a few of the many pain-killing drugs available. To specialised First Aiders, who are likely to have to administer such drugs, I would suggest that they contact a doctor in their own area for further information and advice. In addition, I would advise them most strongly to obtain a legal opinion, BEFORE acquiring any potent drugs.

PRINCIPLES OF TREATMENT OF FRACTURES

The two basic principles of treatment of fractures are:
a. Elimination of shock which involves all three of the basic principles of First Aid (i.e. to preserve life, to prevent deterioration and to promote recovery).
b. Definitive treatment.

a. Elimination of shock

This is vitally important because untreated oligaemic shock (i.e. shock from blood loss) is a potential killer. To this end, it is important to:
 (i) Stop gross bleeding—this minimises the overall blood loss,
 (ii) Administer intravenous fluids—this boosts the circulating blood volume, raises the blood pressure and minimises the depletion of E.C.F. and I.C.F.,
(iii) Institute pain relief (e.g. intramuscular injection of Paraveretum) because pain aggravates shock, and
(iv) Splint adequately because movement at the fracture site causes pain which in turn aggravates shock, and because good splinting minimises the risk of further damage to structures at, or near, the fracture site.

'Adequate' splinting involves immobilisation of the joints above and below the fracture site as well as immobilisation of the fracture site itself. The exact method of splinting of a particular fracture depends upon the equipment at hand (or not at hand as the case may be). If no special equipment is available (e.g. a hare splint), then *ingenuity is the First Aider's best friend*. For instance, a folded newspaper, tied on with string, can form a very adequate U-shaped support for a fractured leg or forearm (but, please remember to support the foot or hand). Prior to splinting, *gross* deformity should be corrected, but please do not re-introduce extruded bone from an open fracture into the wound as this increases greatly the risk of infection.

I have stated many times, and will continue to state, that *methods* of splinting vary according to the type of splints in vogue at different points of time in history, but the *principles* of splinting have remained the same, and will remain the same, throughout history.

b. Definitive treatment

This takes place under the care of hospital personnel whose basic aims are to achieve healing of the fracture (preferably in its original anatomical position) and to restore function. Definitive treatment involves continuation of intravenous fluids until they are no longer needed, manipulation of the fracture under general anaesthetic and fixation of the fracture. Fixation is of two kinds:

(i) External fixation—e.g. Plaster of Paris and various external splints.;

(ii) Internal fixation—this is achieved by open surgery—e.g. a long nail, called a Kuntschner nail, can be passed down the inside of the femur to hold a fractured femoral shaft in perfect position.

Definitive treatment of fractures may also involve surgery to repair tendons, to transplant tendons, or to repair nerves and/or blood vessels. Even plastic surgery can be necessary, after some fractures.

I have purposely avoided a long, classified list of fractures in this book because I wish to stress *principles* rather than detailed facts. For a beautifully concise description of the many different types of fracture, I can do no better than refer the reader to a book called *Outline of Fractures* (1983) by John Crawford Adams, published by Churchill Livingstone, Edinburgh.

12

Chest injuries

I must begin this section with a brief description of the anatomy of the chest, so that confusion can be avoided as you read on. The chest is a bony cage, capable of expansion and contraction. This cage is formed by the ribs, which are attached to the thoracic (or dorsal) vertebrae at the back, and to the sternum (or breastbone) at the front. The ribs afford a certain amount of rigidity to the chest wall and protection for the lungs, whilst at the same time allowing mobility to the chest wall. The gaps between the ribs are filled with muscles, called intercostal muscles, each of which is attached to the rib above and the rib below. In the right side of the chest, there is the right lung and in the left side of the chest, there is the left lung. The lungs are separated from each other by a space which runs down the middle of the chest called the *mediastinum*. This space contains the heart and great arteries and veins, lymph vessels and lymph nodes, trachea (windpipe) oesophagus (gullet), the vagus nerves and sympathetic nerve plexuses. The vagus nerves are cranial nerves (they originate in the brain) and they supply all parts of the alimentary tract. The sympathetic nerve plexuses are part of our autonomic nervous system (the nervous system which functions without our conscious control) and they are found in both thorax and abdomen. Each lung is separated from the chest wall by two layers of *pleura*. One layer of pleura covers the outer surface of the lung and the other layer covers the inner surface of the chest wall. Between the two layers of pleura, there is a thin film of lubricating fluid, so that the two layers of pleura can slide smoothly over each other as the chest expands and contracts.

Landmarks of the chest

At the top of the sternum there is a notch and, quite naturally, it is called the *sternal notch*. This notch lies between the left and right sterno-clavicular joints—the joints formed between the inner ends

142

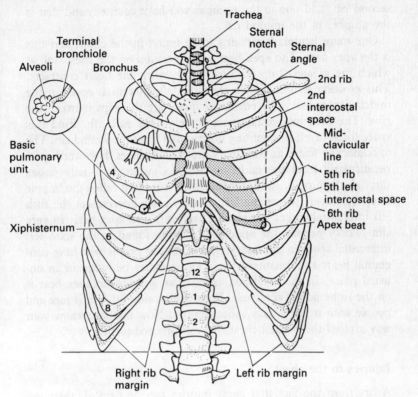

Fig. 34 Landmarks of the chest.

of the clavicles and the sternum. Find your own sternal notch and place the tip of your index finger on top of it. Now, push your finger backwards over the sternal notch, and the tip of your finger will hit your trachea. Normally the trachea is placed centrally behind the sternal notch. Any deviation of the trachea to left or right indicates that something is wrong. Now, run your index finger downwards until you are about one to one-and-a-half inches below the sternal notch. Here, you will feel a ridge running horizontally across the sternum. This ridge is called the *sternal angle*. If you follow the ridge to the left, you will find that it is exactly in line with a rib. This is the *second left rib*. Likewise on the right you will find that the sternal angle is exactly in line with the *second right rib*. By counting downwards from the second rib, on either side you can find the sixth, seventh, eighth, tenth rib etc. If you find a tender rib you can also count upwards from that rib until you reach the second rib, add one to the number you have counted, and that is the number of the injured rib.

One more landmark remains to be found in the chest, and this is the *apex beat*. The apex beat is the position on the chest wall at which the greatest impulse can be felt when the heart contracts. This position is normally in the fifth left intercostal space in the midclavicular line. The *intercostal spaces* are the gaps between the ribs. The fifth intercostal space is below the fifth rib. Find this space for yourself by counting downwards from the second rib. The *midclavicular line* is an imaginary line which passes downwards perpendicularly from the midpoint of the clavicle. It usually passes through the nipple, and for this reason, it is often called the 'nipple line'. However, where the left midclavicular line crosses the fifth left intercostal space, you should find your own apex beat. In very slim, lanky people, the apex beat is often found in the sixth left intercostal space in the midclavicular line. In people who have congenital heart abnormalities, the apex beat may be found in an unusual place. In the condition called *situs inversus* the apex beat is on the right side of the chest. Fortunately, *situs inversus* is rare and people with it are usually quite healthy. Now that you know your way around the normal chest, we can proceed further.

Injuries to the chest

Apart from the fact that chest injuries can be painful, their importance is that they can be detrimental to the general condition of the patient because of:

a. impaired lung function;
b. impaired heart function and
c. blood loss within the chest.

The types of chest injury can be broadly divided into *penetrating* wounds (where a sharp object pierces the chest wall) *blunt* injury (from a blow or fall) and *crushing* injury (if a man is trapped between a wall and a lorry).

A penetrating wound usually causes the lung on the side of the injury to deflate. If the wound is large enough, and it need not be very large, then air will pass through the wound into the chest when the injured person tries to breathe in, and out again when he tries to breathe out. Unfortunately, this can cause the mediastinum to move to-and-fro, from side to side. This movement is known as *mediastinal flap*. It interferes with the function of the heart, causing *cardiogenic shock*, in which the patient is pale and sweating; his blood pressure is low and his pulse is weak and rapid, just as if he had suffered a coronary thrombosis. In fact, it is the same kind of shock as that which occurs in coronary thrombosis. If the patient had some kind of lung disease prior to the collapse of his lung through injury, he would almost certainly show *cyanosis* (blueness of the lips and fingernails), indicating impairment of lung function. Penetrating wounds of the chest can cause bleeding into the chest, but this is not usually very gross. Fortunately, penetrating wounds of the chest are relatively uncommon in peacetime, though they are common in wartime.

Blunt injuries of the chest are by far the commonest seen in peacetime. Someone trips and falls onto his chest, or is thrown onto a steering wheel in a car crash. Crushing injuries are not as common, but they can be as serious, if not more serious, than blunt injuries. The damage sustained from either of these two kinds of injury depends upon the amount of violence involved. The damage ranges from bruised ribs or sternum right through the range of fractured ribs, fractured sternum, bruised heart muscle, bruised lungs and gross bleeding inside the chest, to stove-in-chest. In the stove-in-chest injury, an unstable segment of the chest wall moves inwards as the patient breathes in, and outwards as he breathes out (i.e. in the opposite direction to that in which it should move each time).

This abnormal movement of a segment of the chest wall is called *paradoxical respiration*. It occurs when each of a series of ribs is broken in two places. Paradoxical respiration causes great respiratory distress, mediastinal flap and cardiogenic shock.

A severe blow to the chest (e.g. from a steering wheel in a car crash) can cause *surgical emphysema*. This is a puffy swelling above and behind the clavicles, and when you feel at it, as if playing the piano, it gives the sensation of a soft, crinkly, tissue-paper-like feeling. It is the soft-tissue crepitus to which I referred when I discussed bony crepitus in *injuries to Bones and Joints*. This may not appear for twelve or twenty-four hours after the injury, but if found, it indicates a severe compression injury of the chest. Bleeding inside the chest (between the lungs and the chest wall) after a compression injury may be up to eight pints or more, and blood loss can occur inside the chest whether ribs are fractured or not.

One other injury which I will mention is *ruptured thoracic aorta*. This occurs as the result of a sudden, violent, twisting movement of the trunk. It is usually caused by being thrown from a motor cycle, although it can be caused by a mountaineering accident. The rupture of the aorta may extend down into the abdominal part of the aorta. The condition is usually fatal, unless the patient can be taken to a hospital with a special chest surgical unit. The diagnosis of ruptured thoracic aorta should be suspected.

a. When the history suggests a sudden, violent, twisting movement of the trunk, and

b. When the patient is shocked, in the absence of any other definite signs, or in the presence of relatively minor injuries.

It should also be remembered that an injury to the *lower* ribs may cause damage to organs inside the abdomen. This will be referred to in 'Abdominal Injuries'.

Finally, before we proceed to the examination of the chest, I will remind you that muscle-spasm occurs as a protective mechanism after injury. Just as muscle-spasm after a fracture of the femur can cause a shortening of the femur, so muscle-spasm can reduce the movement of part of the chest wall after injury. The whole object of muscle-spasm after injury is to reduce movement of the injured part to a minimum. This, in turn reduces pain to a minimum. In fact, muscle-spasm is our own built-in, self-splinting mechanism.

Examination of the chest

This is always preceded by the history, of course, and we want to know:

a. How the injury occurred;

b. If the patient is conscious, ask:
   (i) 'Where does it hurt you?' and
   (ii) 'Does it hurt when you take a deep breath?'

c. 'Has there been any previous chest trouble?'

Question (b) (ii) is designed to reveal whether or not a *sharp, stabbing pain* occurs when the patient breathes in, because this is typically the pain which occurs when a rib has been fractured.

Question (c) is a useful one to ask, because if, for example, a man has had one lung removed, then he will tell you right away and this can prevent you from looking foolish later on.

The examination of the chest is where our time-honoured quartet of Inspection, Palpation, Percussion and Auscultation really come into their own.

a. Inspection

First of all, look at the patient's face, whilst feeling at his pulse. This saves time. You can learn very quickly to note the facial appearance, rate and type of respiration, and rate, rhythm and volume of the pulse all in a very short space of time. Make a note of these three things. Next, look at the patient's chest either from directly in front of him or directly behind him, and note whether the chest moves equally when he breathes in and out. If one side of the chest moves *less* than the other, then that side is probably being restricted by muscle-spasm, which indicates a probable injury on that side. Under the heading of Inspection, we can also look for cyanosis.

b. Palpation

First of all feel for the trachea and apex beat. If these are displaced to one side, this may be due to a collapsed lung, or severe bleeding into the chest, or both. We have already 'sprung' the ribs in our initial head-to-toe examination, and we have made a note of any pain so produced. Find any tender rib or ribs, and count up from it or them, as I have already described. Press on the sternum from top to bottom to find if there is any tenderness there. Feel the neck, above and behind the clavicles for surgical emphysema. Make a note of any postive findings, e.g. 'Tender sternum and 5th and 6th left ribs. Surgical emphysema'.

c. Percussion

This is where we drum on the patient's chest.

To practise percussion, place your left middle finger on a table, so that the front of the end *joint* of the finger is pressed firmly against the table. Now, hold your right middle finger in a curved position as if it were a hammer. Then 'drum' or 'hammer' with the tip of your right middle finger on the back of the end joint of the left middle finger, letting the movement flow from the right wrist. By percussing in this way over the middle of the table, you should produce a hollow sound. If you percuss the table-top above one of the legs, you should produce a more solid sound. Percussing a wall, or a stone fireplace should produce an even more solid sound. Having practised percussion on the table, you can now practise it on the front of your chest, and, assuming that you have no gross lung disorder, you should produce a rather hollow note. This is the normal percussion note, and we refer to it as *Resonance*. It varies slightly from one individual to another, depending on the size and shape of the individual chest. When you practise percussion on another person's chest, you should *always* compare one part of the chest with the similar part of the other side—compare upper right front with upper left front and so on.

Hyper-resonance is a much more hollow sound than the normal resonance, and it indicates a collapse of a lung, or part of a lung. When a lung collapses, air is allowed into the pleural cavity, and this is called a *pneumothorax*. Hyper-resonance denotes the presence of a pneumothorax.

Stony dullness is like the note obtained when percussing a stone wall. It indicates fluid in the chest, which, after injury is usually blood. A collection of blood within the chest is called a *Haemothorax*.

d. Auscultation

As I pointed out in Part II, you can hear normal breath sounds, either by placing the ear onto someone else's chest, or by the use of a stethoscope. The breath sounds are heard much more clearly if you ask the patient to breath in and out *through the mouth*. Again, compare upper right front with upper left front, lower right back with lower left back etc. You should listen, also, directly over any tender tibs, because if you hear crepitus (a loud crunching sound), this will confirm your suspicion of a fractured rib.

Let us summarise these steps in the examination of the chest by considering an example. Let us assume that we have found a man who has had a heavy fall onto the left side of the chest. On examination we might well find the following:

1. *Inspection* (General condition and appearance). Face pale; slight cyanosis of lips; cold, clammy skin; rapid thready pulse. These signs indicate
   a. impairment of lung function (because of the cyanosis) and
   b. shock (because of the other signs). Inspection of the chest reveals that the left side of the chest barely moves, indicating that the injury is on the left side.
2. *Palpation.* We find that the left 5th and 6th ribs are tender. We may even feel crepitus as we press on the ribs. Also we find that the trachea and the apex beat are displaced a little to the right.
3. *Percussion.* We find that the percussion note is normal all over the right side of the chest. Over the upper part of the left side of the chest, there is hyper-resonance, and over the lower part of the left side of the chest, there is stony dullness.
4. *Ausculatation.* We find that the breath sounds over the right lung are normal, but the left side of the chest is devoid of breath sounds. We hear crepitus over the 5th and 6th left ribs.

From these findings we conclude that the diagnosis is:
1. Fractured 5th and 6th ribs, left side.
2. Collapsed left lung.
3. Haemothorax, left side (collection of blood).
4. Shock, because of the injuries and the blood loss.

I will leave this example for you to re-ponder, and I will offer you the following two reminders:
a. Hyper-resonance with diminished or absent breath sounds indicates collapsed lung.
b. Stony dullness with diminished or absent breath sounds indicates haemothorax.

Emergency tracheotomy

This is literally a life-saving operation, and it should not be undertaken lightly. Emergency tracheotomy is indicated when the airway is blocked, cannot be unblocked and there is cyanosis. It follows therefore, *that you must make every effort to clear the airway, before embarking on emergency tracheotomy*. Having tried to clear the airway, and having found it impossible to do so, you are left with no alternative but to perform emergency tracheotomy. For this you will need the following:
1. A *sharp* knife.
2. Sharp-pointed scissors.
3. An incompressible tube (preferably curved metal with a guard on one end).
4. The ability to count up to four.
5. COURAGE IN ABUNDANCE!

At a pinch you could manage without the scissors, and instead of a metal tube, you could use (say) the empty barrel of a ball-point pen.

Method. The head and neck must be *fully* extended. To ensure this, place something behind the shoulders to act as a cushion with the patient lying flat. Place a finger on the 'Adam's apple' and slide your finger down the trachea. You will feel rings of cartilage in the trachea, below the 'Adam's apple'. Count your way down these rings until you find the gap between the third and fourth rings. Directly over this space make an incision across the front of the trachea. This incision *must* go through the full thickness of the skin. Having drawn blood, by cutting the skin, this is where you need the 'courage in abundance' to carry on! Either with the knife, or preferably with the *closed* pointed scissors stab between the third and fourth cartilaginous rings. If you have used the scissors, they can be opened to widen the incision through the wall of the trachea, and then can be twisted through a right angle and used in the same way to push the third and fourth rings of cartilage apart and allow the tube to be passed into the trachea. Once the tube has been inserted into the trachea, the scissors can be removed, and the patient should be able to breathe through the tube. The tube should be held in position by the best means available, and the following precautions should be taken:

a. Take care that the patient does not cough out the tube.
b. Take care that no foreign matter (e.g. blood) gets into the tube. A dampened swab over the end of the tube serves as a good filter for this purpose.
c. If possible suck out the tube regularly (if you have a suction apparatus).

I hope that you will never have to perform emergency tracheotomy. However, if you are ever faced with a situation which *demands* tracheotomy, then I hope you will have the courage to do what is necessary to save a life. Otherwise, the patient will surely die.

Some specialised first aiders are now being taught the technique of endotracheal intubation. This technique involves the passing of a lubricated rubber tube into the trachea via the mouth or nose. The part of the tube which enters the trachea, is surrounded by an inflatable cuff. When the tube is in position, the cuff is inflated. The inflated cuff bulges against the wall of the trachea and, therefore it keeps the tube in place, as well as preventing secretions from the nose and mouth from passing into the lungs. Thus, the cuff prevents the unconscious person from drowning in his own secretions, whilst the tube provides a secure airway (N.B. The potential hazards of endotracheal intubation have been stressed already in 'The classical stages of anaesthesia').

Whilst endotracheal intubation can be very useful for dealing with a deeply unconscious person, it is by no means easy and special training is necessary in order to acquire the skill. Also, it *cannot* be used when the airway is blocked and cannot be unblocked. The *only* solution to that problem, as stated previously, is emergency tracheotomy.. This must be performed by the person on the spot. When a person whose airway is blocked and cannot be unblocked begins to show cyanosis (i.e. go blue in the face), then that person has only about ten minutes to live. The only way to save the person's life is to bypass the blockage, by performing an emergency tracheotomy *immediately*, because it may take much longer than ten minutes to summon a doctor to the scene.

SUMMARY OF INJURY AND NON-INJURY CONDITIONS OF THE CHEST

A. INJURY CONDITIONS OF THE CHEST

1. Bruised ribs

History

(i) A blunt injury is described (e.g. a fall or a blow to the chest).
(ii) The patient complains of pain over the affected ribs.

Signs

(i) The affected ribs are tender.
(ii) Breath sounds are normal.
(iii) There is no bony crepitus to be felt or heard.

Treatment

(i) Advise the patient to breathe as normally as possible, support-ing the bruised ribs with hand pressure if necessary.
(ii) Give oral analgesics ('pain-killers') if necessary—e.g. paraceta-mol.

Transport

If it is necessary to transport the patient (e.g. because he has an injured knee as well as the bruised ribs), this should be in the sit-ting position. Otherwise, the patient should be allowed to walk.

2. Bruised sternum

The history, symptoms, signs, treatment and transport are as for bruised ribs, except that it is the sternum which is tender, instead of the ribs.

3. Fractured ribs *(uncomplicated by lung injury)*

History

(i) Blunt injury is described, but greater force is usually involved.
(ii) *Typically*, the patient complains of a *a sharp, stabbing pain on inspiration.*

Signs

(i) Cyanosis is NOT usually observed.
(ii) Restricted movement of the injured side may be observed.
(iii) The affected ribs are tender.
(iv) 'Springing' the chest produces pain at the site (s) of injury.
(v) Breath sounds are normal.
(vi) Audible bony crepitus over the affected ribs *confirms the diagnosis*. (Bony crepitus is often palpable too.)
(vii) Surgical emphysema may be found.

Treatment

(i) Analgesics may be given, but NOT OPIATES (e.g. morphine, papaveretum)
(ii) Lying the patient on the injured side reduces movement of that side which, in turn, reduces pain.

Transport

Preferably, this should be on the injured side, but the sitting position should be used if there is respiratory distress or cyanosis.

4. Fractured sternum

The history, symptoms, signs and treatment are as for a fractured rib, except that the tenderness and bony crepitus are localised to the sternum. Transport can be in the prone position, or, if there is respiratory distress, or cyanosis, in the sitting position.

5. Flail segment

If an injury causes a number of consecutive ribs (say three or more) to fracture, and if each of those ribs is broken in two places, then the middle portions of those ribs can, collectively, form an unstable portion of the chest wall. This is known as a *flail segment* of the chest wall. This flail segment can be splinted by muscle spasm for a few hours after injury, but, when the muscle spasm passes off, the flail segment is then able to move virtually independently of the rest of the chest wall.

Since the act of inspiration creates a decrease in pressure inside the chest, the flail segment is drawn towards the centre of the chest during inspiration whilst the rest of the chest wall is moving away from the centre of the chest. During expiration, the pressure inside the chest is increased. This causes the flail segment to move away from the centre of chest whilst the rest of the chest wall is moving towards the centre of chest. These movements of the flail segment, in the opposite directions to those of the rest of the chest wall, are known as *paradoxical respiration*.

Paradoxical respiration creates pressure differentials between the injured and the uninjured sides of the chest during inspiration and expiration. These pressure differentials cause a side-to-side, to-and-fro movement of the mediastinum which is known as *mediastinal flap*. Since the heart is contained in the mediastinum, mediastinal flap involves movement of the heart from side to side, to and fro, this produces cardiogenic shock.

History

This will describe a very heavy blow to the chest wall.

Signs

  (i) Paradoxical respiration can be seen.
 (ii) There may be cyanosis of the lips.
(iii) Rapid shallow respiration.
 (iv) Shock (i.e. pallor, a cold clammy skin and a rapid thready pulse).
  (v) Lowered blood pressure.

Treatment

  (i) Pack the flail segment in the 'in' position. You cannot stop the flail segment from being drawn inwards, but you can stabilise it by stopping it from coming out again. This will reduce mediastinal flap and cardiogenic shock to a minimum.
 (ii) Lie the injured person on the injured side. This adds to the stabilisation of the flail segment.
(iii) Administer oxygen if there is cyanosis.
 (iv) An intravenous infusion helps to combat shock.
  (v) Avoid administration of opiates unless evacuation is likely to be prolonged (more than six hours) and difficult, or unavoidably rough.

Transport

On the injured side, either recumbent, or semi-recumbent.

6. Sucking (penetrating) wound

When a sharp object penetrates the chest wall and the layer of pleura which covers the inner surface of the chest wall, air can then be drawn into the chest through the penetrating wound during inspiration. This causes the lung on the injured side to collapse. Air can also be expelled through the penetrating wound during expiration. As with flail segment, therefore, pressure differentials are created. During inspiration, the *un*injured lung inflates and the mediastinum is pushed towards the injured side. During expiration, the *un*injured lung deflates and the mediastinum moves towards the uninjured side. In other words, mediastinal flap occurs and, as with flail segment, it causes cardiogenic shock. The other major aggravating factor in this injury is the fact that the whole burden of respiratory function, normally shared by two lungs, is suddenly thrown onto one lung. Haemothorax may occur, either from a punctured lung or from the chest wall wound.

History

This describes a penetrating injury to the chest wall (e.g. by the spike of an ice axe, or by a fall onto a sharp object).

Signs

These are as for flail segment, except that:
  (i) there is no paradoxical respiration,
 (ii) air can be heard to pass into and out of the wound, and
(iii) haemoptysis (coughing up of bright red frothy blood) may occur if the lung on the side of the injury has been punctured.

Treatment

Seal the hole *IMMEDIATELY*. A small sheet of plastic held in place firmly by adhesive strapping is a very useful first aid measure. The strapping should be applied in such a manner that air cannot pass under the edges of the plastic. This will reduce the amount of shock and will also prevent further collapse if the lung not been punctured.

Transport

As for flail segment.

7. Completely obstructed upper airway

This condition is caused most commonly by the inhalation of a foreign body which then blocks the larynx. Sweets and marbles are very often the foreign bodies inhaled by children, whilst pieces of meat and other foods are often the foreign bodies inhaled by adults. Another possible cause of obstructed upper airway is fractured larynx (e.g. from a Karate blow). If the airway is blocked completely, the patient becomes cyanosed very rapidly and unconsciousness supervenes in two minutes. If respiration is not restored within ten minutes at the most, the patient will die from suffocation.

History

This is often accompanied by a great deal of panic! However, verbal expressions such as, 'He can't breathe!', 'He tried to swallow something and it went down the wrong way!', or, 'Something's struck in his throat!', will lead you to suspect the inhalation of a foreign body.

Signs

Initially,
   (i) the patient will be in obvious respiratory distress.
  (ii) the pulse is rapid and bounding.
 (iii) there is cyanosis of the face.
 (iv) the chest moves, in inspiratory efforts, but no air entry is audible through the chest wall (even if the surrounding atmosphere of tumult and panic has given way to one of quiet, morbid curiosity!).
After unconsciousness has supervened,
  (v) the cyanosis deepens until the face appears to be virtually black,
 (vi) the respiratory efforts become progressively weaker.
(vii) the pulse becomes progressively rapid and feeble.
Finally,
(viii) the early signs of death appear (see Diagnosis of death).

Treatment

(i) Removal of the foreign body should be attempted. Various methods have been advocated for this, such as hooking out the foreign body with a finger, a hefty slap on the back, turning the patient upside down, a very rapid 'bear hug' around the lower ribs, or various combinations of these methods. If all efforts to remove the foreign body fail, then the only remaining course of action is to perform

(ii) Emergency tracheotomy (or Cricothyrotomy) to bypass the obstruction. (See 8 (iii) below.)

8. Incompletely obstructed upper airway

This can be caused by *inhalation of a foreign body* which blocks the larynx *in*completely. It can also be caused by *laryngeal oedema* (i.e. soft tissue swelling of the larynx), which, in turn, can be caused by throat infections or by either physical or chemical irritation of the larynx. Chemical irritation, and especially physical irritation of the larynx, can also cause *laryngeal spasm* (i.e. spasm of the vocal cords)—e.g. by trying to pass an endotracheal tube during the second stage of anaesthesia (see Stages of anaesthesia). Laryngeal spasm is occasionally so severe that it blocks the upper airway completely.

Signs

With an incompletely obstructed upper airway, there is obvious respiratory distress and a degree of cyanosis dependent upon the degree of respiratory obstruction; but the most obvious sign is *stridor* (or *laryngeal stridor*). *Stridor* is a high-pitched wound which occurs during inspiration. The patient usually remains conscious

Treatment

(i) Try to remove or expel the foreign body. If this fails,

(ii) Oxygen, if available,should be administered by face-mask.

(iii) Cricothyrotomy may be necessary (i.e. 'needle' tracheotomy).

(iv) Emergency tracheotomy be necessary on the rare occasion when cyanosis deepens, unconsciousness supervenes and there is no improvement after cricothyrotomy.

9. Haemothorax

This is a haematoma (i.e. pool of blood) inside the pleural cavity—i.e. between the lung surface and the chest wall. It may occur as a complication of fractured ribs, ruptured lung or punctured lung. Gravity causes pooling of the blood in the *lower*, posterior part of the chest. It is associated with a collapsed lung on the injured side.

10. Pneumothorax

This is a collection of air in the pleural cavity. It can occur after blunt or penetrating injury. It is usually found in the *upper* part of the chest, on the injured side. It is associated with a collapsed lung on the injured side.

11. Haemopneumothorax

This is a combination of haemothorax and pneumothorax. After chest injury, haemopneumothorax is found much more frequently than haemothorax alone or pneumothorax alone. Haemopneumothorax, of course, is associated with a collapsed lung on the injured side.

Signs

(i) Breathlessness is common.
(ii) Cyanosis is common.
(iii) The injured side of the chest expands less than the uninjured side.
(iv) Hyper-resonance on percussion over the pneumothorax (usually in the upper part of the injured side).
(v) Stony dullness on percussion over the haemothorax (usually in the lower part of the injured side).
(vi) Absent breath sounds over the haemothorax.
(vii) Tenderness will be found over any broken ribs.
(ix) A flail segment may be observed.
(x) A penetrating wound may be observed.

Treatment

(i) Pack a flail segment, if present.
(ii) Seal a penetrating wound, if present.

(iii) Administer oxygen, if available.
(iv) *DO NOT* give morphine or any other opiates because they depress the respiratory centre in the brain.

Transport

Either,   (i) lying on the injured side,
  or, (ii) semi-recumbent but inclined towards the injured side,
  or, (iii) sitting but inclined towards the injured side, whichever is the most comfortable position for the patient.

B. NON-INJURY CONDITIONS OF THE CHEST

1. Spontaneous pneumothorax

This occurs spontaneously, without injury, and is commonly to be found in one side of the upper part of the chest. It is a self-limiting (i.e. non-progressive) condition.

Causes

(i) Spontaneous rupture of a small, congenital abnormality on the surface of the lung (known as a congenital emphysematous bulla) allows air to escape from the lung into the pleural cavity. This is by far the commonest cause these days.

(ii) A number of chest diseases (which need not be listed here) can cause spontaneous pneumothorax. For example, rupture of a lung surface affected by tuberculosis *was* the commonest cause of spontaneous pneumothorax up to the early and mid-twentieth century. Thanks to the advent of better treatment and control of tuberculosis this is now a rare cause of spontaneous pneumothorax.

Symptoms

A sudden sharp pain, followed by a continuous dull ache in the upper part of the chest.
The signs, treatment and transport are as for traumatic pneumothorax.

2. Tension pneumothorax

This is a progressive form of pneumothorax, in which the amount of air inside the pleural cavity increases gradually. The rupture of the lung surface produces a flap-valve effect. This allows air to pass from the lung into the pleural cavity as the flap-valve opens during inspiration. On expiration, the flap-valve closes, preventing the return of air from the pleural cavity to the lung. Thus, the air in the pleural cavity increases in quantity with every inspiratory effort. The increasing quantity of air in the pleural cavity exerts an ever increasing pressure upon the affected lung, collapsing it and gradually pushing it towards the healthy side of the chest. If this process is allowed to continue, the ever-increasing pressure exerts its effect on the heart, gradually reducing the ability of the ventricles to fill. Cardiac output is reduced progressively until unconsciousness supervenes because insufficient oxygenated blood is reaching the brain. About ten to twenty minutes after unconsciousness occurs, the patient dies because of severe cerebral hypoxia.

Symptoms and signs

As for spontaneous pneumothorax, but with the addition of ever-increasing breathlessness and cyanosis, together with the appearance of the signs of cardiogenic shock (pallor, cold clammy skin and a rapid thready pulse).

Treatment

(i) Oxygen by mask is a very useful initial measure.
(ii) The main aim is to reduce the pressure in the pleural cavity, or at least to prevent further increase in pressure. This can be achieved by pushing a fairly wide-bore needle through the chest wall of the affected side, just above the third rib, in the mid-clavicular ('nipple') line. When the tip of the needle enters the pleural cavity, a hissing sound is heard as the air rushes out through the needle. The hissing sound stops when the pressure in the pleural cavity equals atmospheric pressure. The needle should be held in position by adhesive tape.
It is important to understand that, by penetrating the chest wall, a *sucking wound* has been created. Therefore, if the flow of air through the needle is not regulated, *mediastinal flap* and *cardiogenic shock* can ensue. These can be prevented by using a

thumb to block the end of the needle every time the patient breathes in, and releasing the blockage every time the patient breathes out. This prevents the entry of air into the pleural cavity via the chest wall during inspiration. A small amount of air will enter the pleural cavity via the flap-valve defect in the surface of the lung during each inspiration, but the same amount of air will leave the pleural cavity via the needle during each expiration. The overall effect of this technique is to place a second flap valve into the system, so that the flap-valve defect in the lung surface allows air into the pleural cavity on inspiration, and the 'thumb and needle' flap-valve allows the same quantity of air to leave the pleural cavity on expiration. The patient's chest condition thus becomes stabilised, as does his general condition.

A special needle has, in fact, been developed with a built-in flap-valve effect. This releases one person from the obligation of performing the 'thumb and needle' technique constantly until the patient can be handed over to medical care.

Transport

(i) In the sitting position, once the chest and general conditions have been stabilised. The carry should be as comfortable as possible.

(ii) DO NOT give opiates (e.g. morphine).

(iii) If the patient's general condition is quite good, or if the diagnosis could be spontaneous pneumothorax as opposed to tension pneumothorax, it may be deemed adequate simply to transport the patient to hospital in the sitting position without inserting a needle into the chest. However, if the general condition deteriorates, and especially if unconsciousness supervenes, the transport must be stopped. When a needle has been inserted into the chest and when the patient's general condition has improved (i.e. consciousness has been recovered and signs of shock, breathlessness and cyanosis have passed away), then the transportation may be resumed.

3. Bronchial asthma (often referred to simply as 'Asthma').

Causes

These are numerous: many allergies can cause asthma, notably allergy to house dust and the house dust mites and hay fever. Some pharmacological products produce asthma in susceptible people. Psychological factors may be the cause. Even exercise can produce asthma in some people (i.e. exercise-induced asthma).

Mechanism

Bronchospasm occurs. This is really a spasm or narrowing of the *bronchioles* rather than of the bronchi. Therefore, it would be more correctly termed bronchiolar spasm. However, bronchospasm is a narrowing of the bronchioles, and when it occurs, air passes more easily into the alveoli than it can pass out again. Thus, the patient tends to take in more air than he expels, gradually accumulating air in the lungs until he is breathing with his lungs virtually fully inflated all the time. At this stage, he can be seen to be using his *accessory muscles of respiration* (i.e. the neck muscles and muscles around the upper chest are seen to tense up on inspiration). These accessory muscles of respiration are used to pull the upper part of the chest upwards and outwards in order to attain the fullest possible capacity of the lungs.

Signs.

  (i) Obvious breathlessness.
 (ii) Sweating.
(iii) Pulse rapid and bounding.
 (iv) Accessory muscles of respiration in action.
  (v) *Expiratory* rhonchi can be heard, i.e. 'wheezing', but only as the patient breathes *out* (of Bronchitis—see below).
 (vi) Cyanosis may be present.

Treatment

  (i) Allow the patient to use his usual treatment (e.g. an inhaler) if it is available.
 (ii) Tell him to concentrate on breathing out as far as he can each time he breathes out.
(iii) The paper bag method of treatment can be very useful. Inflate a paper or plastic bag and place it over the patient's nose and mouth so that the seal is airtight. The patient then breathes the same air in and out continuously. This leads to a build-up of carbon dioxide content in the rebreathed air, and the in-

creasing intake of carbon dioxide provides a good stimulus to the respiratory centre in the brain. This method is often successful in increasing expiratory effort and producing relaxation of the bronchioles.

(iv) Oxygen by mask is sometimes helpful.

(v) Further treatment of bronchial asthma lies outside the scope of the First Aider; though, in the U.S.A. a doctor may instruct a paramedic by radio to give certain drugs intravenously.

Transport

Preferably sitting.

4. Cardiac asthma

Causes

This occurs because of Left Ventricular Failure (ref. L.V.F., i.e. inefficient function of the left ventricle of the heart). A number of medical conditions, notably valvular disease of the heart and myocardial infarction, can cause L.V.F., but it can occur also in climbers at high altitudes.

Signs

(i) Severe breathlessness. Typically, the affected person wakes up in the early hours of the morning gasping for air. This is known as Paroxysmal Nocturnal Dyspnoea (ref. P.N.D.).

(ii) Pallor

(iii) Sweating ⎫ i.e. signs of cardio-

(iv) Rapid and rather feeble pulse ⎭ genic shock.

(v) Crepitations (moist, bubbly sounds) are heard at the lung bases (i.e. at each side of the lower part of the back of the chest).

Treatment

(i) Sit the patient up.

(ii) Administer oxygen, if available.

N.B. Opiates—e.g. papaveretum ('Omnopon') or morphine—can be very helpful in the treatment of L.V.F., but should *not* be given to a person who is suffering from valvular heart disease, particularly mitral stenosis. Therefore, if there is any doubt at all, a medically qualified person should decide whether or not to use opiates. Similarly, the decision to use, or not to use, a diuretic should be the responsibility of a medically qualified person. Diuretics are drugs which increase output of urine. This reduces the total amount of fluid in the body which, in turn, relieves the pulmonary oedema (excess fluid) in the lung bases.

Transport

In the sitting position.

5. Myocardial infarction (coronary thrombosis)

Cause

The blood supply to part of the heart muscle becomes blocked off and the part of the heart muscle which is deprived of blood supply, dies.

Symptoms

Typically, the patient experiences a severe 'crushing' pain across the front of the chest. The pain usually radiates down the left upper limb, but it may also radiate down both upper limbs or just down the right upper limb.

Signs

The signs are those of cardiogenic shock, namely:

(i) Pallor
(ii) Cold, clammy skin
(iii) Rapid, feeble pulse, although sometimes the pulse may be *slow* if the patient has gone into heart block.
(iv) Reduced blood pressure. (*N.B. A person displaying the foregoing symptoms and signs may have a blood pressure of, say, 130/80, which, in normal circumstances, could well be accepted as a normal blood pressure. However, his blood pressure prior to the occurrence of the infarct could well have been 180/110. Therefore, the diagnosis should be made on the basis of the other symptoms and signs. The blood pressure readings should be taken to obtain a baseline and to monitor the patient's progress.*)

Treatment

(i) Sit, or lie, in the most comfortable position for the patient.
(ii) Oxygen, if available, should be administered, especially (but not only) to cyanosed patients.
(iii) A strong analgesic (e.g. papaveretum) should be given intra-muscularly, or intravenously, if a doctor is present and deems it desirable.
(iv) *WAIT* for the analgesic to take effect. Even if you have to wait twenty or thirty minutes, the patient will be in a much better general condition for transporting to hospital than he would be whilst still shocked and in pain.

Transport

(i) To hospital, gently and smoothly, in the position which is most comfortable for the patient, monitoring the pulse and blood pressure.
(ii) If cardiac arrest occurs, stop the transport (unless he is already in an ambulance) and commence cardio-pulmonary resuscitation (C.P.R.) immediately.

6. Bronchitis
Causes

This is a condition in which thick mucus adheres to the inner surfaces of the bronchi and bronchioles. It may result from infections, especially virus infections, or it may be caused by chemical irritation.

Signs

(i) Productive cough (i.e. the patient coughs up sputum).
(ii) Breathlessness, even at rest.
(iii) Cyanosis may be present, depending upon the previous condition of the lungs and upon how many of the bronchioles are blocked.
(iv) *Inspiratory* rhonchi (wheezes) can be heard on auscultation (cf bronchial asthma).

Treatment

(i) Oxygen should be administered if the patient is markedly cyanosed.
(ii) Otherwise, refer him to his doctor.

7. Tracheitis

Causes

This is an inflammatory condition of the inner surface of the trachea ('windpipe'). It can arise after a sore throat, common cold, or influenza. It may also be caused by chemical irritation.

Symptoms

(i) Typically, the patient complains of a severe burning sensation behind the breast bone, especially on breathing in rapidly or on coughing.
(ii) General malaise (i.e. feeling generally unwell).

Signs

(i) The patient may appear unwell.
(ii) Dry, unproductive cough (i.e. does not cough up sputum initially, although some sputum may be coughed up after a few days as the illness is overcome.
(iii) Otherwise, there is usually very little to find.

Treatment

Refer to a doctor.

8. Pleurisy

Causes

This is an infection near the surface of a lung which causes inflammation of the pleura. The smooth nature of the pleura covering the affected part of the lung is lost and, therefore, smooth movement is lost, as the pleura covering the lung slides over the pleura covering the inside of the chest wall. Rough jerky movement between the two layers of pleura occurs, and this rough, jerky movement causes pain in the part of the chest wall covering the infected area. After about three days, the affected layers of pleura pour out fluid. The fluid separates the affected layers of pleura, and this eliminates the rough, jerky movement between them. Therefore, the pain ceases. Pleurisy often follows a sore throat, common cold, or influenza.

Symptoms

The patient:
   (i) complains of a sharp stabbing pain, especially on inspiration. (The pain is localised to the affected area.)
  (ii) feels generally ill (general malaise).
 (iii) may admit to having had a sore throat, cold, or influenza, in the previous week or two.

Signs

   (i) Looks ill.
  (ii) Inspiration is obviously painful (i.e. the patient winces).
 (iii) Restricted chest movement on the affected side.
  (iv) Pulse is often rapid and bounding.
   (v) Temperature is usually markedly raised.
  (vi) A *pleural rub* is audible over the site of the pain. This is a coarse, grating sound.

Treatment

Lie the patient on the affected side, semi-recumbent if necessary.

Transport

In this position to hospital or to the nearest doctor: or summon the doctor to the patient if the patient is at home.

9. Pneumonia

Causes

This may follow a throat infection, or may occur as a primary infection.

Symptoms

   (i) General malaise.
  (ii) Weakness.

Signs

   (i) The patient looks ill (pale or flushed).
  (ii) There may be a tinge of cyanosis of the lips.

(iii) Increased rate and depth of respiration.
(iv) Pulse rapid and bounding.
 (v) Rigors occur—i.e. shivering attacks.
(vi) The temperature is raised.
(vii) Dilirium may occur (e.g. he may see people who are not there).
(viii) Unconsciousness may supervene.
(ix) Rales (rather coarse, bubbly sounds) may be heard all over the lungs.

N.B. In the very old, chest movements are often so restricted that no abnormal sounds can be heard in the chest, yet most of the other signs (except (iii) above) will be present. Chest infection is a notable cause of dilirium in the elderly.

Treatment

Administer oxygen, if available.

Transport

In the sitting, or semi-recumbent position.

10. Lobar pneumonia

Causes

This is a condition in which invading organisms infect one lobe of a lung, usually a lower lobe. These organisms produce toxins (poisons) which are very dangerous to human beings. In the days before sulphonamides and antibiotics were available, it was quite common for a young and hitherto healthy person to contract lobar pneumonia, to be unconscious within six hours and dead within twelve hours of contracting the disease. Antibiotics now give us a good chance of overcoming this condition, but, because of the extremely rapid nature of its progress, *lobar pneumonia is still a potential killer.*

Signs

 (i) Facial appearance—looks ill, face very flushed and dry, initially; later, may develop pallor and sweating as pulse begins to fail.
 (ii) Pulse—initially, rapid and bounding; later, fades to rapid and thready.

(iii) Rigors occur (i.e. shivering bouts).
(iv) Respiration—initially, increased in rate and depth; later, decreased rate and depth; may proceed to Cheyne-Stokes respiration terminally (i.e. just before death).
 (v) Rales (sometimes with rhonchi) are audible over the affected lobe of the lung.
(vi) Some dullness is usually detectable over the affected lobe of the lung.
(vii) Temperature–raised; often up to 105°F (about 40.5°C).
(viii) If untreated, the patient loses consciousness and a crisis ensues. following which:
    a. he dies quite rapidly, or
    b. the temperature falls dramatically and recovery commences.

Treatment

Administer oxygen, if available.

Transport

 (i) In sitting position, if conscious, or
(ii) In the recovery position, lying on the affected side, if unconscious.

11. Hysterical hyperventillation

Description

This is a condition in which the patient actively overbreathes, or hyperventillates his lungs, and which can be brought on by a host of psychological factors. This hyperventillation may cause a claw-like spasm of the hands and forearms, known as tetanic spasm.

Explanation of tetanic spasm (N.B. Those, who find this explanation too technical, should ignore it and pass on to the treatment!). The blood contains a certain amount of carbon dioxide which is being carried to the lungs by haemoglobin in the red blood cells, but a considerable quantity of carbon dioxide dissolves in the blood's fluid and forms carbonic acid which separates into hydrogen ions and bicarbonate ions. The bicarbonate ions form an important part of the blood's chemical buffer system which is important in maintaining the acid/base balance of the blood. If a person hyperventillates (overbreathes), carbon dioxide can be expired via the lungs at an excessive rate. This can deplete the bicarbonate ions in the blood, which disturbs the acid/base balance of the blood.

Calcium in the blood and tissue fluids is in two forms, i.e. (a) free calcium ions and (b) protein-bound calcium. If muscles are to relax properly after contracting, a certain amount of free calcium ions in the nerve and muscle tissues is essential. A marked reduction of bicarbonate ions, such as that which can be caused by hyperventillation, results in a marked reduction of free calcium ions and an increase in protein-bound calcium. This, in turn, results in muscular spasm which really is a loss of the ability of the muscles to relax.

Treatment

(i) If the patient is out of danger, persuade him to lie down, cover him with a blanket and leave him *'severely'* alone for about half an hour. *Attention prolongs the condition.* The less fuss and bother, the sooner the patient will recover his composure.

(ii) If the patient is in a dangerous position (e.g. a climber who suddenly experiences an extreme fear of falling, or a person on a ledge on the outside of a high building), then different tactics must be adopted. It should be remembered that shouting angrily at the patient or ridiculing him will only worsen matters. The rescuer must speak calmly and give any instructions confidently and with an air of authority—e.g. 'Don't move. I'm coming to help you. I'll get you out of here safely.' Please, *never* use the expression 'Don't panic!', because the very mention of the word 'panic' is virtually bound to increase his already-existing state of panic!

If our patient on the high building can be encouraged to keep still, then there is an excellent chance of reaching him, securing him and assisting him to safety, but beware of those last few feet to the patient. This is the time when he will feel a desperate need to grab for his rescuer. If he attempts this, he may fall to his death. Therefore, the rescuer must carry on talking, making it quite plain that the patient must stay still and that he (the rescuer) will come to the patient.

In some climbing situations, it is not feasible for a rescuer to approach the patient. Therefore, if he cannot be persuaded to continue the climb, it may be necessary for his colleagues to haul him up by his safety rope which is used by most modern climbers. (I use the word 'colleagues' and not, 'colleague', because it is very difficult, if not impossible, for one person to haul up another person bodily on a climbing rope, or on any other kind of rope, for that matter.)

12. Exertional tachycardia

Increase in heart rate occurs in fit people on exertion, but they do not suffer from it. Exertional tachycardia means rapid beating of the heart which occurs in *unfit* people who over-exert themselves, trying to keep pace with fitter companions.

Symptoms

(i) Breathlessness.
(ii) Extreme lassitude (fatigue).
(iii) Palpitations (or 'fluttering' in the chest).

Signs

(i) Breathlessness.
(ii) Pallor.
(iii) Sweating (often profuse).
(iv) The patient may fall to the ground, exhausted.
(v) Very rapid pulse (often in the 180 to 200 per minute range).

Treatment

(i) Rest and reassurance.
(ii) Slow down the pace of the fitter companions.

Transport

Usually quite unnecessary.

13. Paroxysmal tachycardia (paroxysmal ventricular tachycardia)

This condition should not be confused with exertional tachycardia. It occurs in people who are usually quite healthy, and the patient is often an otherwise fit young man, to whom the condition is no more than a nuisance. The patient suddenly experiences a fluttering sensation (i.e. tachycardia) in the chest, which stops him in his tracks. This lasts for only a few seconds, after which the patient feels perfectly well and able to continue his activities immediately. The tachycardia may occur at rest. It tends to recur at irregular intervals and without warning. It is not accompanied by pain. The patient learns to live with the condition.

Symptoms and signs

(i) The patient suddenly stands still or sits still and stops talking.
(ii) There is no alteration in facial colour as a rule.
(iii) The patient admits to palpitations or 'flutterings', if questioned.
(iv) The patient may volunteer, or admit to, previous similar episodes.
(v) The pulse is very rapid, during the attack, but normal afterwards.

Treatment

Allow the patient to rest for a few seconds until the tachycardia has passed off spontaneously.

Transport

Not necessary. The heart rate returns to normal in a few seconds, and the patient feels quite well immediately.

13

Abdominal injuries

Penetrating injuries of the abdomen are uncommon in peacetime, but are common in wartime, and they may cause injury to any organ inside the abdomen. *Closed injuries* of the abdomen are far more likely to occur in peacetime. The organs most commonly damaged are the liver, spleen, kidneys, bladder and urethra (the tube through which urine flows from the bladder to the outside world). These organs are the ones most commonly injured, because they are relatively immobile within the abdomen. The stomach and intestines usually escape injury from a blow to the abdomen, because they are relatively mobile within the abdomen. It has been said that the rectum may be torn in association with a nasty pelvic fracture, but quite frankly it is a very rare occurrence.

The liver, spleen and kidneys are tucked away neatly in the upper part of the abdomen. They lie below the diaphragm, which separates the chest from the abdomen, and they are hidden by the lower ribs, with the exception of about the lower two thirds of each kidney. *The kidneys* lie in the loins at the back of the upper abdomen, and they cannot normally be felt. *The spleen* is about one-and-a-half times the size of a fist, and normally it cannot be felt as it is hidden by the left lower ribs. Similarly, the bulk of the *liver* is protected by the right lower ribs, and so the liver cannot normally be felt. However, by pressing under the right rib margin at the front of the abdomen, you may elicit tenderness which in turn would make you suspect a rupture of the liver. Similarly, pressure under the left rib margin at the front of the abdomen could elicit tenderness, which would raise your suspicion of a ruptured spleen. If, by pressing in the left loin, you were to find tenderness, you would suspect a ruptured left kidney. If you found tenderness in the right loin, you would suspect a ruptured right kidney. *The urethra* is attached fairly firmly to the lower surface of the pubic bone, which you can feel at the middle of the front of the lower end of the abdomen and which is part of the pelvis. For this reason, the

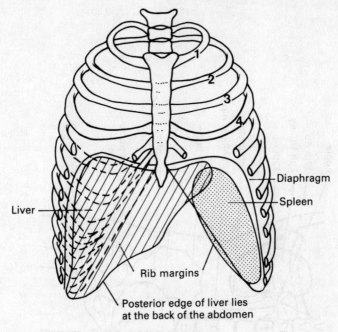

Fig. 35 Location of liver and spleen (front view).

urethra is more often injured than the *bladder* which lies in the 'pit' of the stomach, behind the pubic bone. The bladder is relatively fixed within the abdomen by virtue of the fact that it is necessarily attached to the urethra, which is attached to the pubic bone. A full bladder is more likely to be injured than an empty one, because the wall of the bladder is held in a more rigid state when the bladder is full, than when it is empty. You will not be able to feel an empty bladder, though you may be able to feel a full one. Tenderness in the abdomen, just above the pubic bone, indicates the probability of a ruptured bladder. Blood in the urine usually comes from a ruptured urethra though it may also come from a ruptured bladder.

As in other parts of the body, muscle-spasm occurs in the abdomen as a built-in splinting mechanism after injury. *Rigidity* is the term we use to describe muscle-spasm of the abdominal wall. Rigidity occurs because bleeding inside the abdomen irritates the peritoneum, which is the sensitive inner lining of the abdomen. *Guarding* is the term used to describe the involuntary tensing of the patient's abdominal muscles in response to quite gentle pressure over the site of tenderness. After a fall onto the back, bleeding can

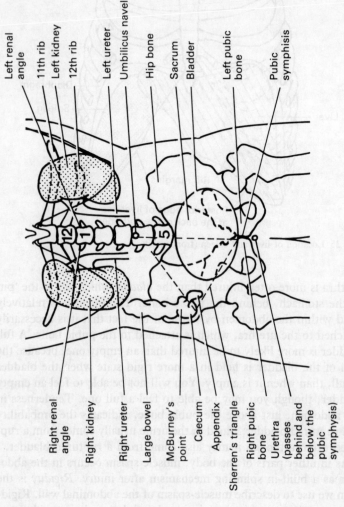

Left renal angle
11th rib
Left kidney
12th rib
Left ureter
Umbilicus navel
Hip bone
Sacrum
Bladder
Left pubic bone
Pubic symphisis

Right renal angle
Right kidney
Right ureter
McBurney's point
Caecum
Appendix
Sherren's triangle
Right pubic bone
Urethra (passes behind and below the pubic symphysis)

Fig. 36 Location of kidneys, ureters, bladder, urethra and appendix.

occur from the muscles which cover the front of the lower thoracic and lumbar vertebrae and a collection of blood forms in front of those muscles and behind the peritoneum which covers the back of the abdomen. Such a collection of blood is called a *retroperitoneal haematoma* (retro—behind; peritoneal—referring to the peritoneum; haematoma—a collection of blood in an abnormal situation). A retroperitoneal haematoma can account for two to four pints of blood-loss. Therefore, it should be borne in mind as a possible diagnosis if you are confronted with a man who has fallen onto his back, is in shock and has generalised rigidity of the abdomen, in the absence of any other definite signs or obviously serious injury (compare this with ruptured thoracic aorta described in *Chest injuries*).

The following points are useful to remember when dealing with someone who may have a closed abdominal injury:

1. Visible bruising on the abdominal wall almost always indicates internal injury.

2. A fall onto the left lower ribs may damage the spleen or the left kidney.

3. A fall onto the right lower ribs may damage the liver or the right kidney.

4. A fall onto the back may damage the right or left kidney, or it may cause a retroperitoneal haematoma.

5. An injury to the pelvis may damage the urethra or bladder.

6. Absent bowel sounds, in the presence of abdominal tenderness and rigidity (especially if the patient is shocked) indicate internal injury. Absent bowel sounds, *without* abdominal tenderness etc. can occur after severe blood-loss, or immediately after being concussed.

7. Blood loss from internal abdominal injuries can be *catastrophic*. Hence the importance of suspecting and detecting abdominal injuries before it is too late and the patient dies pouring out blood internally. It is also important to satisfy yourself that a person has NOT sustained an abdominal injury, because that is one injury less to worry about.

8. A person with a damaged spleen may be standing or walking about when you first see him. Do not let the 'walking casualty' fool you into neglecting to examine his abdomen. To do so could result in his death!

I shall never forget the day when I was shown an X-ray film of the left ribs of an eighteen-year-old boy. I could see no fractures on the X-ray film, so I went to the boy and asked him what had happened. He said that he was a railway worker and that he had been walking along a railway track and had slipped. As he fell, his left lower ribs had landed heavily on one of the railway lines. His face was rather pale and on examination I found rigidity down the left side of the abdomen, tenderness under the left rib margin and absent bowel sounds. I had no hesitation in diagnosing a ruptured spleen, even though he had walked into the accident department. His spleen was removed forthwith, and I trust that he will live to a ripe old age.

History

When asking the patient how the injury happened, you should be trying to create a mental picture of the accident—the way in which he fell and how he landed (remember: 'The words, 'I fell' should ring a bell'). You should also ask him to show you where he feels pain and you should ask him whether or not he has had any abdominal operations. Make a note of his answers.

Examination of the abdomen

Once again our time-honoured quartet goes into action:

a. Inspection

(1) Assess his general condition by looking at his face, feeling the pulse and taking the blood pressure. It is important to record the blood pressure if at all possible.

(2) Look for visible signs of bruising on the abdominal wall.

(3) See whether the abdomen moves with respiration, which is normal, or if it is held rigidly, which is abnormal.

b. Palpation

(1) Make sure that your hands are warm, as cold hands will cause the abdominal muscles to tighten up.

(2) Slide your hand *gently* around the abdomen. Only in this way will you be able to feel *rigidity* if it is present in any part of the abdominal wall.

(3) Ask the patient to breathe deeply and slowly through the mouth. As he breathes out his abdomen will be as relaxed as it possibly can be.

(4) Press gently but firmly all over the abdomen to elicit tenderness. Also try to push your finger ends under each rib margin. Do not forget to press in the loins below the ribs at the back to elicit kidney tenderness.

(5) If you find tenderness, tell the patient to tighten his abdominal muscles and then press again. *If it hurts more* when you press on his tensed abdomen, then the tenderness is caused by bruising of the muscles of the abdominal wall. *If it hurts less* then the tenderness is inside the abdomen itself.

(6) Tell him to breathe deeply again, and then test all over the front of the abdomen for *rebound tenderness*. To do this, press down firmly and slowly, then suddenly release your pressure. If this causes pain and a sudden contraction of the abdominal muscles which makes the patient wince, then that is rebound tenderness. It is caused by irritation of the peritoneum by bleeding. Bleeding inside the abdomen can track downwards, and so it is quite common to find tenderness under the rib margin and rigidity and rebound tenderness lower down the abdomen, but on the same side.

c. Percussion

In examining the abdomen, the First Aider can percuss over the lower part of the abdomen. If the bladder is full, then the area of the lower abdomen which covers the bladder will give a dull note, compared with the rest of the abdomen, which will give a drum-like, or 'tympanitic' note. If the bladder is empty, the whole of the abdomen should give a tympanitic note. Apart from this, percussion of the abdomen is not a great deal of help to the First Aider, and further discussion of it would only serve to confuse him.

d. Auscultation

At the start of the Part I, I told you to listen to bowel sounds by placing your ear against someone else's abdomen. So you should be able to recognise normal bowel sounds by now! When bleeding occurs inside the abdomen, it irritates the intestines. This causes the irritated segment of bowel to try to empty itself and so, at first you may hear *hurried* bowel sounds (i.e. bowel sounds occurring in quicker succession than normally). You may hear the odd *gurgling* sound at this stage too. Later when the bowel segment has almost emptied itself, slow, *tinkling* bowel sounds can be heard. Finally, when the bowel segment is empty, it ceases all movement and at this stage, no bowel sounds can be heard. The bowel sounds are said to be *absent*.

Let us now imagine that we are examining a man who has fallen onto his back. We find that his face is pale, his skin dry, his pulse bounding and his blood pressure is $\frac{160}{90}$ (i.e. he is displaying the 'adrenaline response', at this stage). We see that his abdomen is held rather rigidly and, on palpation we find tenderness in the right loin, and rigidity and rebound tenderness down the right side of the abdomen. After percussing the lower abdomen, we decide that the bladder is empty and on auscultation, we find that the bowel sounds are absent. The diagnosis which *must* be suspected here is that of *ruptured right kidney*, and that diagnosis stands until the abdominal surgeons prove otherwise. The patient should be taken to hospital as soon as possible, because once his adrenaline response passes off, his blood pressure could collapse dramatically, with dire consequences for the patient.

Please practise examination of the abdomen. It is important
   a. to exclude abdominal injury, if there is none present, and
   b. to find an abdominal injury, if one exists.

You cannot hope to find abdominal injuries unless you look, feel and listen to the abdomen.

SUMMARY OF INJURY AND NON-INJURY CONDITIONS OF THE ABDOMEN

A. INJURY CONDITIONS OF THE ABDOMEN

1. Ruptured gut

This is caused usually by penetrating injury—e.g. from a knife, or an ice axe.

Signs

  (i) There is often a visible wound of the abdominal wall.
 (ii) The signs of shock are present (pallor, cold clammy skin and a rapid thready pulse), because of damage to the sensitive peritoneum which lines the inner surface of the abdominal wall.
(iii) Rigidity, guarding, tenderness and rebound tenderness occur. Initially, these signs are localised to the site of the injury. Later, they may become generalised if peritonitis develops,

because of spillage of unsterile gut contents into the normally sterile abdominal cavity.

(iv) The bowel sounds are hurried at first. Later, they are tinkling, and later still they are absent.

Treatment

(i) Keep the patient warm.

(ii) An intravenous infusion helps to combat shock.

(iii) Monitor the vital signs regularly (pulse, respiration and blood pressure, in particular).

(iv) If any gut is protruding, DO NOT ATTEMPT TO PUSH IT BACK! (That would introduce infectious organisms into the abdominal cavity which would cause peritonitis.) Simply cover the gut with a warm, damp and preferably sterile cloth.

(v) Transport the patient to hospital lying flat on his back unless he has lost consciousness, in which case, use the recovery position.

(vi) Avoid giving the patient analgesics *unless* the evacuation route is so long and arduous that evacuation is likely to take six hours or more.

2. Ruptured spleen

This is caused usually by blunt injury (e.g. a fall)

Signs

(i) The signs of shock are present.

(ii) There is tenderness *under* the left rib margin.

(iii) Guarding, rigidity and rebound tenderness occur *below* the left rib margin, and they may extend down the *left* side of the abdomen.

(iv) Bowel sounds are diminished or absent.

Treatment

As for ruptured gut (with the exception of the warm, damp cloth, of course!)

N.B. Delayed rupture of the spleen can occur up to fourteen days after blunt injury because the capsule of the spleen may not be ruptured immediately, even though the pulp, which lies inside the capsule, may be ruptured at injury. Eventually, the capsule gives way, the signs of ruptured spleen ensue, and blood loss can be catastrophic. For this reason, a person with *suspected* rupture of the spleen should be observed in hospital for up to fourteen days. Delayed rupture of the spleen should be suspected if the history is suggestive, the patient's face is pale (even without the full signs of shock) and if there is tenderness under the rib margin.

3. Ruptured liver

This is caused by both blunt and penetrating injuries. As in the case of the spleen, delayed rupture of the liver can occur up to fourteen days after blunt injury.

Signs

As for ruptured spleen, but the signs are on the *right* side of the abdomen.

Treatment and transport

As for ruptured spleen.

4. Ruptured right kidney

This is caused usually by blunt injury.

Signs

(i) Shock.
(ii) Tenderness in the right loin.
(iii) Rigidity, guarding and tenderness may develop down the right side of the front of the abdomen.
(iv) Bowel sounds are diminished or absent.

Treatment and transport

As for ruptured spleen.

5. Ruptured left kidney

As for ruptured right kidney, but the signs are on the left.

6. Ruptured bladder

This is caused usually by blunt injury; it is often associated with a fractured pelvis. A full bladder is more likely to be ruptured by injury to the lower abdomen than is an empty bladder.

Signs

  (i) Shock.
 (ii) Tenderness in the middle of the lower abdomen (just above the pubis).
(iii) Rigidity, guarding and rebound tenderness occur at the site of the tenderness.
 (iv) These signs extend laterally to right and left across the lower abdomen, initially. Later, they tend to extend towards the upper abdomen.
  (v) Bowel sounds are diminished or absent.
 (vi) The urine, if any is voided, contains blood.
(vii) There may also be signs of a fractured pelvis.

Treatment and transport

As for ruptured spleen, but a fractured pelvis (even a stable fracture) should be well padded.

7. Ruptured urethra

This is very commonly associated with a fractured pelvis.

Signs

  (i) Shock.
 (ii) The urine, if any is voided, contains blood.
(iii) Signs of fractured pelvis are commonly in evidence.

Treatment and transport

As for ruptured bladder.

8. Retroperitoneal haematoma

This can be caused by a heavy blow, either to the lumbar region or to the front of the abdomen. Bleeding occurs, either from a fractured vertebra or from the muscles which lie in front of the spine, and a haematoma forms in front of those muscles and behind the peritoneum which covers the posterior abdominal wall; hence, 'retro- (=behind) peritoneal haematoma.' The haematoma may contain 1–2 litres (2–4 pints) of blood.

Signs

  (i) Shock.
 (ii) *Generalised* abdominal tenderness.
(iii) The abdominal wall may feel distended and rather tense.
(iv) Bowel sounds are absent.

Treatment and transport

As for ruptured spleen.

B. NON-INJURY CONDITIONS OF THE ABDOMEN

1. Gastroenteritis

This is an inflammatory condition of the stomach and intestines, in which a great deal of fluid can be lost because of diarrhoea and vomiting.

Causes

These are numerous and include virus infections (e.g. influenzal gastroenteritis), typhoid, paratyphoid A, paratyphoid B, cholera and botulism (which is usually fatal).

Symptoms

General malaise; colicky pains which move all over the abdomen; diarrhoea and vomiting.

Signs

  (i) Pallor.
 (ii) Prostration.
(iii) Rapid, bounding pulse.
(iv) Diarrhoea.

(v) Vomiting.

(vi) Absence of rigidity, guarding, tenderness and rebound tenderness.

(vii) Hurried bowel sounds.

(viii) Signs of shock supervene later if fluid loss is not corrected.

Treatment

(i) Antiemetic (i.e. a drug to stop vomiting).

(ii) Fluid replacement—orally; or by intravenous drip if necessary.

(iii) Antidiarrhoeal (i.e. drug to stop diarrhoea).

Transport

In the recovery position if vomiting has not stopped completely, otherwise, lying flat and facing upwards.

2. Acute appendicitis (acute inflammation of the appendix)

Symptoms

(i) General malaise (i.e. the patient feels generally unwell).

(ii) Waves of nausea, associated with:

(iii) Colicky, central abdominal pains (i.e. across the umbilicus). A colicky pain is one which commences, increases gradually to a maximum intensity and then fades away gradually, i.e. it produces a crescendo of pain.

(iv) After about six hours, the colicky pains settle in (i.e. are confined to) the right iliac fossa (i.e. the pain becomes localised to McBurney's point).

(v) *Typically*, the patient vomits *once only*. Occasionally, vomiting is recurrent.

(vi) In acute retrocaecal appendicitis (i.e. when the appendix lies behind the first part of the large bowel, which is the caecum and therefore is in contact with the muscle which covers the inner aspect of the hip bone), there is pain in the right buttock, though the buttock is not tender.

Signs

(i) The patient looks pale and ill.

(ii) The pulse is usually rapid and bounding

(iii) There is rigidity over the right iliac fossa.

(iv) Guarding, tenderness and rebound tenderness are found over McBurney's point (see Fig. 36).

(v) Cross-rebound tenderness is present—i.e. on testing for rebound tenderness in the *left* iliac fossa, the patient experiences pain in the *right* iliac fossa.

(vi) There is hyperaesthesia of Sherren's triangle (i.e. there is *increased sensitivity* to light touch over Sherren's triangle compared with the left side of the lower abdomen). This can be tested by stroking each side of the lower abdomen, in turn, using a piece of cotton wool, a small finely-bristled brush, or the tip of a finger.

Treatment

'The treatment for acute appendicitis is appendicectomy.' (Here, I quote numerous surgeons, past and present!)

Transport

Keep the patient warm and transport him to hospital, either lying on his back, or (if he still feels sick) in the *right* recovery position.

3. Acute Meckel's diverticulitis

Meckel's diverticulum is a small sac which protrudes from the ileum (the last part of the small bowel). It occurs in two per cent of people, is about two centimeters (four fifths of an inch) long and is found about two feet away from the appendix, as one traces backwards along the ileum from its junction with the large bowel. Like the appendix, Meckel's diverticulum can become inflamed.

Symptoms and signs

These are as for acute appendicitis, except that the pains settle in the *left* iliac fossa where the signs are also to be found (e.g. tenderness).

Treatment and transport

Again, these are as for acute appendicitis, except that the *left* recovery position should be used, if the patient still feels sick.

4. Duodenal ulcer

This is a small ulcer in the duodenum. The duodenum is the first part of the small bowel and food passes into it from the stomach. If the ulcer is *active*, there are symptoms; if it is *inactive*, there are no symptoms. Typically, a person who has a duodenal ulcer suffers symptoms for a few weeks at a time, during which periods the ulcer is active. In between such periods, the person is symptomless.

Symptoms

(i) Indigestion (i.e. pain). This occurs in the upper central part of the abdomen (epigastrium—see Fig. 14.0), or sometimes a little lower. It occurs particularly if a meal is overdue, and it tends to waken the patient at night. The pain is eased by food, milk drinks, or antacid tablets and mixtures. It is aggravated by fatty foods, spicey foods, spirits, smoking, worry and overwork.

(ii) Weight gain occurs, because of eating to releave symptoms.

(iii) Eructation occurs (i.e. bringing up wind, or 'belching'.)

(iv) Waterbrash may occur (i.e. regurgitation of gastric juice).

Signs

(i) The 'pointing' sign is positive—i.e. if asked to show where he feels the pain, he will point *with one finger* to the exact spot, instead of placing his flat hand over it. This spot is in the *right* epigastrium.

(ii) Guarding and tenderness are found in the *right* epigastrium.

(iii) Intermittent borborygmi ('gurgling sounds') can be heard, below and lateral to the site of tenderness, signifying duodenal 'hurry' as food passes through the duodenum.

Treatment

(i) Avoid aggravating factors.

(ii) Regular meals and a regulated life-style (shift work is bad for 'D.U.s').

(iii) Antacids, as necessary.

5. Perforated duodenal ulcer

This is fairly common, and 20 per cent of perforated duodenal ulcers occur without the patient having had any previous appreciable symptoms of duodenal ulcer.

Symptoms

(i) Sudden onset of severe, colicky, upper abdominal pain.
(ii) Previous history suggestive of duodenal ulcer, in 80 per cent of cases.
(iii) Vomiting is quite common.

Signs

(i) Shock is common.
(ii) *Board-like abdominal rigidity* is typical. The whole abdomen feels as hard as a board.
(iii) Tenderness and rebound tenderness are found in the *right* epigastrium and they may extend down the *right* side of the abdomen.
(iv) Bowel sounds disappear quite quickly, leaving the typical sign of *absent bowel sounds*.

Treatment and transport

(i) The patient must be taken to hospital at once. He, or she, should be transported face upward, or in the *right* recovery position, if still vomiting.
(ii) An anti-emetic (anti-vomiting drug) can be helpful.
(iii) An intravenous infusion helps to combat shock.

N.B. (i) Duodenal ulcer and perforated duodenal ulcer can occur virtually at any age. It is a common fallacy that only adults can be affected. I have seen a six-year old boy who was recovering from an operation to repair a perforated duodenal ulcer! In general practice, I have discovered a number of children, some of them only four years old, who have duodenal ulcers, and X-ray evidence has confirmed the vast majority of these cases. Even those whose ulcers are too small to be confirmed by X-rays, have responded well to appropriate treatment.

(ii) Duodenal ulcers are never malignant.

6. Gastric ulcer

This is an ulcer in the stomach. It may be active, or inactive. Periods of activity tend to be quite prolonged. *A minority* of gastric ulcers are malignant.

Symptoms

(i) Indigestion. This occurs typically just after a meal and often is not relieved by antacids.
(ii) Vomiting after meals is common.
(iii) Weight-loss (because of vomiting undigested food) is typical.
(iv) Eractation and waterbrash are less common than with duodenal ulcer.

Signs

(i) The 'pointing sign' is negative. The patient uses a flat hand to demonstrate a vague and poorly localised site of pain.
(ii) Guarding and tenderness are found in the *left* epigastrium.
(iii) Bowel sounds are usually normal.

Treatment

(i) There is no first aid treatment other than administration of what has been prescribed by the patient's doctor.
(ii) Refer to a doctor if the patient has not consulted one already.

7. Perforated gastric ulcer

This is much less common than perforated duodenal ulcer.

Symptoms and signs

These are similar to those of a perforated duodenal ulcer, except that:
(i) The previous history suggests gastric ulcer.
(ii) There is not quite a board-like rigidity of the abdomen.
(iii) Tenderness and rebound tenderness are found usually in the *left* epigastrium and they may extend down the *left* side of the abdomen.

Treatment and transport

As for perforated duodenal ulcer, but in the *left* recovery position, if necessary.

8. Haematemesis

This means vomiting of blood. Duodenal ulcers and gastric ulcers are the main causes, although, once upon an examination time, a very bright, final-year medical student listed one hundred and twenty-one possible causes of haematemesis. So, anyone who really wants to know the other one hundred and nineteen possible causes should consult a very bright, final year medical student!

Symptoms

Vomiting of blood, with or without a previous history of duodenal or gastric ulcer.

Signs

(i) Fresh or slightly darkened blood visible as vomitus.
(ii) Signs of shock may be present, depending on the volume of blood lost.
(iii) Signs of duodenal or gastric ulcer may be evident.

Treatment

(i) An anti-emetic may be helpful.
(ii) An intravenous infusion helps to combat shock (especially a blood transfusion).
(iii) If shock is severe, papaveretum is very helpful.

Transport

In the *right* recovery position if there is danger of further vomiting.

9. Maleana

This is blood which is passed in the stools, but which has come from a bleeding point fairly high up the alimentary tract (e.g. from a duodenal ulcer). During its passage through the gut, the blood is acted upon by digestive enzymes so that when it is finally passed in the stools it has a shiny, *jet-black* appearance. This is in contrast with the bright red blood, which can be lost from haemorrhoids (piles) (N.B. Non-shiny, black stools can result from taking iron tablets, but they are *not* jet-black. Their colour is more like that of a pencil-lead.) Maleana also has a characteristic odour.

Symptoms

(i) General malaise.
(ii) There may be abdominal pain, or there may be no pain at all.
(iii) Passing *jet-black* stools. (N.B. This symptom is not always volunteered by the patient. Therefore, if in doubt, *ASK!*)

Signs

(i) Shock.
(ii) There may be abdominal tenderness.
(iii) Maleana may be visible.

Treatment

(i) An intravenous infusion, especially of blood, can combat shock.
(ii) Papaveretum may be very helpful for severe shock.

Transport

The patient may be transported to hospital lying flat on his back.

10. Haematemesis and malaena

Yes, they can occur together, commonly from a duodenal ulcer. The symptoms, signs, treatment and transport are a combination of those just described for the two conditions individually.

11. Hernia

This is a protrusion of part of the abdominal contents (often a segment of gut or even part of the bladder) through a weakness which is usually in the abdominal wall, although internal herniae are possible (i.e. inside the abdomen). The common herniae occur in the groin where they often can be seen or felt as lumps. If the hernia can be reduced (i.e. pushed back into the abdomen), then the problem is one of nuisance value only. If the hernia becomes wedged in the opening through which it has emerged, and if it cannot be reduced, then it becomes a *strangulated hernia*, with the constriction at the opening causing complete cessation of blood supply to the contents of the hernia. This constitutes an *abdominal emergency* for which the patient requires urgent surgery.

Symptoms and signs

Commonly, there is a sudden onset of central abdominal pain and vomiting, with pain at the site of the strangulation. A tender, tense, irreducible, soft-tissue swelling is found in the groin, and bowel sounds are usually absent.

Treatment

Immediate admission to a surgical unit is essential.

Transport

In the recovery position because of danger of inhalation of vomitus.

N.B. Strangulated parumbilical hernia is one which occurs to one side of the umbilicus. Apart from the fact that the tender, irreducible swelling is near the umbilicus, the symptoms, signs, treatment and transport are as for the strangulated herniae in the groin.

There are numerous other conditions which constitute abdominal emergencies. They need not be listed here because usually the patient is so obviously ill and the condition so obviously abdominal in origin that the only course open to First Aiders is to seek medical aid as quickly as possible.

14

Pregnancy

Most books on First Aid describe 'Emergency Childbirth', but I have not yet found one which tries to improve the First Aider's knowledge of pregnancy. As a result of this, when confronted with a pregnant woman who has injured a limb, the First Aider tends, at best to feel lost and at worst, to feel panic, often when there is no need for either. The object of this Subject is to give the First Aider confidence through knowledge and to enable him to reassure the pregnant woman with a limb injury that her pregnancy is still intact. After all, it should be remembered that the human race has been reproducing itself for about half a million years, and pregnancy and labour are normal parts of the process of reproduction. It is true that doctors and midwives see pregnant women regularly at antenatal clinics, but in the majority of cases, their function is to reassure themselves and the mother-to-be that everything is proceeding *normally*. Similarly, during labour, the function of the doctors and midwives is to supervise labour in order to see that it is proceeding *normally*, and to intervene *only* in the few cases which do not go according to plan. Therefore, the first thing for the First Aider to learn is that pregnancy and labour are normal events in the calendar of human life, and that, in the vast majority of cases— Nature knows best!

General information about pregnancy

The average duration of pregnancy is forty weeks which is ten *lunar* months or two hundred and eighty days or approximately nine calendar months and one week. A useful point to remember is that three calendar months (e.g. from 15th June to 15th September) are thirteen weeks, roughly. Therefore nine calendar months are equal to thirty-nine weeks. The date on which the baby is due to be born is called the expected date of confinement (EDC) or the expected date of delivery (EDD). This is calculated as being forty weeks after the *first* day of the last *normal* menstrual period. I stress the word 'normal' because it is quite common for a 'period' to occur after conception has taken place, but this period is not a normal one because it is usually of shorter duration than a normal period and it usually occurs later than a normal period would be expected to occur. In actual practice we calculate the EDC by taking the date on which the last normal period began, adding seven days and then adding nine calendar months (or subtracting three calendar months, which gives the same answer). For example:

	Example 1	*Example 2*
First day of last period	1st September	30th September
Add seven days	8th September	7th October
Add nine months	8th June	7th July
EDC	8th June	7th July

When the pregnant woman reaches her EDC she is said to be *at term*. After conception, the fertilised ovum is implanted into the inner lining of the womb, and at the site of implantation the 'after-birth' or *placenta* develops. The placenta is essential for the survival of the unborn baby, because the baby is being incubated inside a sac of fluid within the mother's womb and therefore it cannot breathe in the normal way, nor can it forage for food. The baby is isolated in the fluid (liquor) contained in the bag of *membranes*. The baby's blood flows along the umbilical cord from the baby to the placenta, and then back to the baby. Likewise, the mother's blood flows through cavities in the wall of the womb next to the placenta. In this way oxygen and foodstuffs can pass from the mother's blood to the baby's blood through the placenta, and carbon dioxide and other excretory products pass from the baby's blood to the mother's blood. The placenta does not allow the mother's blood to mix with the baby's blood, because this could be disastrous for the baby, especially if its blood group were different from the mother's blood group. The baby is, then, entirely dependent upon the mother and the placenta for survival. If the placenta becomes detached completely from the wall of the womb, the baby will die by suffocation, because it will have lost its supply of oxygen.

The womb grows in size as pregnancy continues and at term, it is a large, powerful, muscular organ, ready to expel the baby during labour. During the last twelve weeks of pregnancy the mother feels the womb contract from time to time, but these are not painful contractions. They are known as Braxton-Hicks contractions, and they indicate that the womb is toning itself up in preparation for the hard work it will have to do during labour, when the force of its contraction reaches up to fifty pounds per square inch. I often wonder how babies survive such a force, but in fact they do. The womb provides protection for the growing baby, since any shock waves are dispersed through the liquor inside the womb. The womb also acts as an incubator for the baby and if a woman is in premature labour, the best baby-incubator in the world for transporting the baby to hospital is the womb itself.

As pregnancy advances, the baby grows steadily bigger. A woman who is having her first baby will feel *movements* any time from the twentieth week onwards (usually about the twenty-fourth week). These movements are caused by the baby's arms and legs as it moves itself about inside the womb. A woman who is having a second or third baby may feel these movements any time from the sixteenth week of pregnancy onwards. At twenty weeks the fundus (i.e. upper end of the womb) is up to the level of the navel, and the fundus can be found by pressing with the edge of the palm. If you begin near the top of the abdomen and then move your palm a little further down the abdomen before you press again, eventually by repeating this action, you will find the fundus. At the twenty-eighth week of pregnancy the fundus is about half way between the navel and the lower end of the sternum. At term it is up to the lower end of the sternum. If you are lucky enough to find a pregnant woman who will let you feel at her abdomen, then take the opportunity to do so (suitably chaperoned of course!), because such opportunities will not arise often for the First Aider. Similarly, if you have the chance to listen to an unborn baby's heart, then take it. The heart can usually be heard best by placing your ear to the mother's abdomen, either in the left lower or right lower part of the abdomen, depending on which way the baby is lying. The baby's heart can be heard faintly at twenty-eight weeks and as term is approached it becomes louder, and therefore much easier to hear. Its rate is about one hundred and twenty beats a minute.

If the baby is born before the thirty-fifth week of pregnancy its chances of survival are rather poor. From the thirty-fifth week up to the thirty-eighth week there is a sharp improvement in the survival rate. From the thirty-eighth week right through to the forty-second week the survival rate is the same—i.e. the baby has the same chance of survival whether it is born two weeks prematurely,

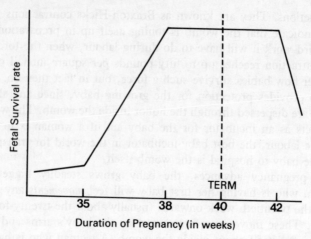

Fig. 37

two weeks overdue, or at term. If pregnancy continues beyond forty-two weeks the placenta begins to degenerate and the baby's chances of survival begin to fall quite sharply. Legally, an unborn baby is deemed to be capable of a separate, independent existence from the end of the twenty-eight week of pregnancy onwards. We use this feature of the law to define abortion (commonly called 'miscarriage') and premature labour, as follows:

Abortion is defined as 'the expulsion of the products of conception (i.e. the baby and the placenta) *before* the end of the twenty-eighth week of pregnancy'. Abortion is the correct medical term for miscarriage. It should not be confused with *criminal* abortion, nor with legal termination of pregnancy.

Premature labour is defined as 'expulsion of the products of conception *after* the end of the twenty-eighth week of pregnancy and *before* term'.

The legal importance of these two definitions is that, when an abortion occurs there is no need to obtain a death certificate for the baby. However, when premature labour occurs and the baby dies, it is necessary by law, to obtain a death certificate for the baby, otherwise the person, or persons, concerned may be charged with *Concealment of birth* (under the law of England and Wales) or with either *Concealment of pregnancy* or *Child murder* (under Scottish Law). These are all serious offences.

Let us now consider Labour, Premature labour and Abortion, in that order.

Labour

In Britain, 80 per cent, or more, of babies are born in hospital, and the arrangements for hospital delivery are usually made well in advance of labour. There is no doubt in my mind that the safest place for any woman in labour is a proper maternity unit of a hospital. Therefore the first sensible thing to do for any woman at term and in labour is to warn the appropriate maternity unit (i.e. the one where she has been booked for confinement) by telephone so that the unit will prepare for her arrival. The second sensible thing to do is to get her to the unit as quickly and *safely* as possible. If the woman is booked for home confinement, she will be able to give you the telephone number of the midwife on call. If a woman is not booked for home or hospital confinement, then this means that she has not attended antenatal clinic as she should have done, and she is a very foolish woman indeed. Nevertheless, under these circumstances, the correct procedure is to contact the general practitioner on call, because he can arrange for her admission to hospital.

It would seem that I have left the First Aider very little to do, but it could happen that a First Aider arrives on the scene just as delivery of the baby is imminent and there is no time to take the mother to hospital. On a number of occasions it has happened that a baby has been born in an ambulance on the way to hospital, with an ambulanceman acting as midwife. So it will do you no harm to know what is going on during labour.

We can divide labour up into three stages. *The First Stage* of labour is that in which the neck of the womb is dilating, and the baby's head is being pushed steadily down into the pelvis. It may last for a few hours. *The Second Stage* is that in which the baby is pushed out (born) and it begins when the neck of the womb is *fully* dilated. This stage normally lasts for no more than one hour, although it may last for as little as ten minutes, especially if the woman has had babies previously. *The Third Stage* is that in which the placenta and membranes are delivered. Since it follows the birth of the baby, it explains why the placenta is often called the 'afterbirth'. This stage may be completed a few minutes after the second stage, or it may last up to an hour. You must *never* interfere with it or you may cause very severe bleeding. Having gained the basic information about labour, we can now consider each of the three stages of labour in rather more detail.

THE FIRST STAGE of labour begins with irregular, sharp, abdominal pains, sometimes accompanied by low backache. The mother passes a small amount of blood-stained mucus from the vagina and this blood-stained mucus is called a *Show*. The mucus has been released from the neck of the womb, where it has been acting as a barrier to keep out infectious germs during pregnancy. Every time the womb contracts, the mother feels a pain. If you place a hand on her abdomen you can actually feel the womb tighten up and relax, as the contraction builds up and as it passes off. The contractions (and the pains, too) gradually become stronger and last longer. The pattern of the contractions changes gradually from an irregular one to a regular one in which the contractions occur about every ten minutes. When this point is reached, the first stage of labour is said to be *established*. From this point onwards the contractions increase steadily in strength, frequency and duration.

As previously stated, these contractions serve to push the baby's head firmly into the pelvis and to dilate the neck of the womb. They also cause the membranes to bulge increasingly through the ever-widening neck of the womb, and eventually the membranes rupture, liberating a sudden gush of crystal-clear liquor. When this gush of liquor occurs you know that *the membranes have ruptured*. This may happen late on in the first stage or it may be delayed until the second stage of labour. When a woman is having her first baby it is quite common for the first stage to last twelve hours or more. Women who have had babies previously, tend to have shorter first stages and second stages too.

Actions in first stage

1. Encourage the woman to conserve her energy, because she will need it during the second stage. You can do this by:

    a. Telling her to relax between pains, by breathing slowly.

    b. Telling her to pant deeply and rapidly whenever she has a pain. This will help her to relax with pains.

    c. Telling her not to push in the first stage, because this will sap her strength and it could be positively harmful to her.

2. Fluid refreshment should be given but NOT solid food.

3. Every fifteen minutes record the time interval, in minutes, between the beginning of one contraction and the beginning of the next. For example, if this time interval is ten minutes, we would record it as 'contractions 1:10'. If it were six minutes we would record it as 'contractions 1:6.' This record not only provides us with a useful indication of the way in which the first stage is progressing,

but it also shows the mother that she is not being neglected!

4. Record the time at which the Show is passed. If the Show was passed before you arrived on the scene, ask the mother when it was passed.

5. Record the time at which the membranes rupture.

THE SECOND STAGE of labour may last up to one hour, or it may be finished in ten minutes or less. It begins when the neck of the womb is *fully dilated* and this is indicated by:

1. very strong pains occurring every three minutes, and

2. an *irresistible* urge to push, felt by the mother, with each pain.

The mother is compelled to push with each pain, and gradually the baby's head becomes visible. When the widest part of the baby's head has reached the outlet of the vagina, the head is said to be *crowned*. Next, the rest of the head emerges, and having done so, the baby's head turns, so that it comes to face either directly to the mother's right side, or directly to the mother's left side, depending on the position of the baby's body, which is still inside the womb. It will be appreciated that, if the baby is facing to the mother's right side, the baby's right shoulder will lie towards the front of the mother and its left shoulder will lie towards the back of the mother. In this case, the right shoulder is said to be the *anterior shoulder*, i.e. the shoulder which is lying towards the anterior part (front part) of the mother. If the baby is facing towards the mother's left side, then the reverse is the case and the left shoulder is the anterior shoulder. It is important to ensure that the anterior shoulder is delivered before the other shoulder, otherwise the mother could sustain a rather bad vaginal tear. Once the anterior shoulder has emerged, the rest of the baby's body slips out quite easily. After the whole of the baby has been delivered, the umbilical cord continues to pulsate for about a minute or so. This pulsation can be felt by holding the cord *gently* between your thumb and fingers. When the cord stops pulsating, this marks the end of the second stage of labour.

Actions in second stage

1. When the mother feels a pain coming on, tell her to take a deep breath, hold it and push hard while the pain lasts.

2. Between pains, encourage the mother to relax as much as possible.

3. As the head of the baby crowns, tell the mother 'Don't push! Pant as hard as you can!' At the same time place your hand against

the baby's head to guard against sudden expulsion of the head. If the baby's head is expelled suddenly, the mother may tear herself, and the baby could suffer brain damage.

4. The next move is to deliver the rest of the baby's head *between contractions* (between one pain and the next). So, when the head is crowned, and when the mother has panted until the pain has passed away, tell her to give a *gentle* push, whilst you are still exerting counter-pressure with your hand. This will allow the head to emerge gently, and the mother should sustain no more than a slight tear of the vagina. In fact, she will probably escape without a tear at all.

5. FEEL FOR THE CORD! This is very important. As soon as all of the baby's head has emerged, feel around the baby's neck for the cord, which may be wrapped around the baby's neck and which could strangle the baby as the rest of the baby is born. Therefore:

a. If the cord cannot be felt, you breathe freely and wait for the next pain.

b. If the cord is around the neck, hook a finger round it and pull until there is sufficient play in the cord to unwrap it from around the baby's neck.

c. If the cord is wrapped so tightly round the baby's neck that you cannot unwrap it, it must be ligated, divided and then unwrapped. To do this, select one part of the cord, slip two ligatures around it and tie them *tightly* about one inch from each other (shoe laces will do for ligatures). Next, cut the cord between the two ligatures, *taking care* not to cut any other part of the cord, or the baby's neck or face. The cord will now easily unwrap from the baby's neck. Should you have to ligate and divide the cord, it is important that the mother does not push until it has been done. Therefore, you must tell her to 'pant like mad' if she feels a pain, and not to push until you have ligated, divided and unwrapped the cord. You should complete this task with all possible speed, because the mother's patience and endurance of pain are both being stretched to the limit at this stage in the proceedings.

6. *With the next pain*, the anterior shoulder should be delivered. To do this, tell the mother to push and at the same time you should exert very *gentle* traction on the baby's head and neck. This traction should be exerted downwards and backwards in relation to the mother (i.e. downwards towards her feet and backwards towards her sacrum).

7. Once the anterior shoulder has emerged, cease the traction

and allow the rest of the baby's body to slide out under the force of the mother's push. *The baby is now born. Make a note of the time of birth.*

8. Now, hold the baby upside down to allow any liquor and secretions to drain out of the mouth. The baby should begin to breathe and cry spontaneously. If necessary, smack it on the bottom to make it cry.

9. *When the cord stops pulsating* tie two ligatures *firmly* around the cord about one inch apart and a good six inches from the baby's navel area. Then divide the cord between the two ligatures. If you have had to divide the cord already (as in 5 c.) simply make sure that you tie a firm ligature six inches away from the baby.

10. Wrap the baby snuggly in a towel or a baby blanket, and then put the baby to the mother's breast. Putting the baby to the mother's breast does three things. First it pleases the mother and the sight of her baby gives her a sense of achievement at the end of her pregnancy. Secondly, it is comforting to the baby and gives it a feeling of security. Thirdly when the baby suckles on the mother's breast, it stimulates chemical activity within the mother, which tones up the womb for further contractions which cause expulsion of the placenta.

THE THIRD STAGE OF LABOUR commences when the cord has stopped pulsating, and it ends when the placenta and membranes have been expelled *completely*. This stage commonly lasts half-an-hour, although it may be as little as ten minutes, or up to an hour. After expulsion of the baby, the womb takes a well deserved rest, and it is important that you allow the womb to rest. In third stage the golden rule is NO UNNECESSARY INTERFERENCE. I cannot stress this too strongly because third stage interference is the greatest cause of third stage haemorrhage! So, be patient and let Nature take its course.

It will be appreciated that, once the womb has expelled the baby, it will contract down because it has emptied itself of a large proportion of its burden. The fundus of the womb should now be just below the level of the mother's navel, and it should feel firm. Having satisfied yourself of this, *keep your hands off the fundus!* You will also realise that the part of the cord which is still attached to the placenta, is visible at the vagina from which it is protruding. We now wait for the *three signs of separation of the placenta*, which are:
a. the fundus rises
b. the cord lengthens
c. fresh bleeding occurs from the vagina

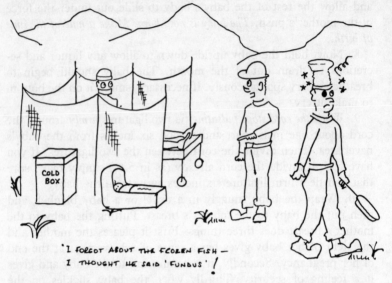

'I FORGOT ABOUT THE FROZEN FISH —
I THOUGHT HE SAID 'FUNDUS'!

Fig. 38 Hands off the fundus

a. The fundus of the womb rises and falls repeatedly, but the general trend is for the fundus to move upwards towards the navel. This causes bleeding to occur between the placenta and the wall of the womb, which separates the placenta from the wall of the womb.

b. As the placenta is pushed downwards within the womb, so more of the cord emerges from the vagina, causing an increase in the length of the cord outside the vagina.

c. The fresh bleeding comes from the bleeding which separates the placenta from the wall of the womb.

When these three signs occur, they indicate placental separation. As they occur, the mother feels another pain in her abdomen and the desire to push returns. As she pushes, she expels the placenta, membranes and blood, and after this the womb contracts down firmly and the bleeding stops. Labour is now finished. It is normal to lose up to one pint of blood during third stage, but more than one pint of blood-loss is abnormal. For this reason, it is important to have some form of receptacle in which the blood can be collected as it leaves the vagina so that the amount of blood lost can be measured. The placenta and membranes are usually collected in the same receptacle and it is important to preserve them, so that a doctor or midwife can inspect them later to ensure that they have expelled completely. If part of the placenta or membranes have been retained inside the womb, secondary haemorrhage may occur later on, or infection may supervene after a few days. So, preserve the placenta for inspection.

Actions in third stage

1. Wait. NO UNNECESSARY INTERFERENCE! I re-emphasise this.
2. Watch for the signs of placental separation.
3. Have a receptacle ready to receive the placenta, membranes and blood.
4. After the mother has pushed out the placenta and membranes, *feel for the fundus*. The fundus should be about half way between the navel and the pubic bone and it should feel firm.
5. Preserve the placenta and membranes for inspection (preferably in a plastic bag).
6. Measure the amount of blood lost. If you cannot measure it then preserve it for measurement later on.
7. Make a note of the time the placenta and membranes were expelled.
8. Tell the mother to cross her legs. This restricts any oozing of blood from a vaginal tear, if she has sustained one.
9. Ensure that the mother is warm and comfortable (and baby too.)
10. Brew up! Mother has earned a nice cup of tea —and so have you! In any case, the mother should not be moved for at least an hour after the end of third stage, and one or two cups of tea help to replace the volume of blood lost during third stage, apart from making her feel refreshed.

I hope that you can now understand what goes on during a normal labour and I hope that you realise that there is nothing very terrible about being at a normal delivery. After all, it is the mother who does all the hard work! What she needs most of all from you is encouragement, confidence and reassurance. If you find the foregoing description of labour and its management too hard to remember, then just remember the following important points:

1. Give the mother encouragement and reassurance.
2. No pushing in First Stage. Mother must pant with pains.
3. Encourage mother to push with pains in Second Stage.
4. The baby's head must be delivered *between* contractions (i.e. between pains).
5. *Feel for the cord* as soon as the baby's head is delivered.

6. The baby's body must be delivered *with* a contraction and NEVER between contractions. If you deliver the body between contractions, you may cause serious, even fatal, bleeding from the womb.

7. Wait for the signs of placental separation. No interference in Third Stage.

8. Collect and preserve the placenta, membranes and blood.

9. Keep mother and baby warm and comfortable after delivery.

10. Brew up the tea. You must not forget that!

Premature labour

More often than not, premature labour occurs for no obvious reason. Occasionally, it occurs because of weakness of the neck of the womb. Sometimes spontaneous bleeding occurs between the placenta and the wall of the womb causing separation of part, or all, of the placenta from the wall of the womb. Such spontaneous bleeding is called *Accidental haemorrhage*, although it usually occurs spontaneously and *not* because of injury sustained by the mother. In fact, although I have seen many pregnant women who have fallen downstairs, or who have been involved in road accidents, I have seen only one woman who, by falling directly onto her abdomen, had caused separation of the placenta and hence the death of her baby. As I stated previously, the womb affords the baby great protection and although many pregnant women sustain injuries by falling, the vast majority of unborn babies come to no harm whatsoever.

On the stage, on television and in films, it quite often happens that 'our heroine' loses her baby as a result of falling downstairs. In real life this is a very rare occurrence indeed, even if the mother does fall downstairs.

Accidental haemorrhage, then, is spontaneous bleeding between the placenta and the wall of the womb. It causes muscle-spasm in the wall of the womb at the site of the bleeding and if you press on that part of the womb, you will find tenderness, though the rest of the womb will not be tender. As you might expect, accidental haemorrhage can trigger off premature labour.

The last cause of premature labour which I will mention is the death of the unborn baby (the technical term for this is *'fetal death in utero'* or FDIU for brevity). If for any reason the unborn baby dies in the womb, its death is soon followed by the onset of labour, presumably because there is no future in incubating a dead baby.

The signs of FDIU are:
1. the womb ceases to increase in size as it normally does during pregnancy.
2. the mother ceases to feel movements and
3. the baby's heartbeat can no longer be heard.

The symptoms, signs and stages of premature labour follow roughly the same pattern as those of labour at term, except that where premature labour has been brought on by accidental haemorrhage, the first symptom may be a severe pain localised to one part of the womb and the first signs may be vaginal bleeding (from the haemorrhage inside the womb) associated with localised tenderness and rigidity of one part of the womb. Usually, the baby is delivered before the placenta, but in premature labour sometimes the placenta may be delivered before the baby, in which case the baby will be stillborn. Blood loss in premature labour is not usually severe, but occasionally it can be.

Actions in premature labour

The mother must be taken to a hospital which has a Premature Baby Unit, where incubators are available for premature babies. No matter how far on in labour the mother appears to be, her womb is still the best incubator in which to take the baby to hospital. If you can contact her doctor first, do so, because he will arrange for her admission in the correct manner. However, if you are way out in the wilds of nowhere, just strap the mother to a stretcher and get moving! If the baby happens to be born on the way to hospital, wrap it up and keep it as warm as you can. Do not forget to ligate and divide the cord and preserve the placenta and membranes for inspection, if they are expelled.

Abortion (Miscarriage)

About one pregnancy in five ends as an abortion and it is usually found to be due to the fact that there was some fault in the fertilised ovum, which would have resulted in some serious defect in the baby had the pregnancy continued to term. No blame can be attached to the parents for the fault in the fertilised ovum. It just happens that these faults occur from time to time because human reproduction is not one hundred percent perfect. We can regard spontaneous abortion as Nature's way of filtering out the defects during the early part of pregnancy, rather than allowing the human defects to be born at term with little or no chance of survival. It is true that some babies are born with defects of the heart, brain, limbs, nervous system etc., but the fact that the vast majority of human beings are born in perfect health shows just how well Nature's filtering system works.

Symptoms of abortion

These may commence in any order. They are:

a. *Vaginal bleeding*. This is often the first sign. It may be very slight at first and then become heavier. The mother often passes clots of blood and in all, abortion may result in the loss of a few pints of blood.

b. *A 'fleshy' substance* may be passed, often with the clots of blood. You should ask the mother if she has passed a fleshy substance. If she has, then it should be retained for inspection if it is still available, because this fleshly substance is probably the *ovum*.

c. *Low backache*. This is often quite severe and it may be the first symptom.

d. *Low abdominal pains*. If the woman has had a baby previously, she will tell you that these pains are like labour pains, and in fact they are caused by contractions of the womb. The pains become regular and they increase in strength and frequency, just like labour pains.

Signs of abortion

a. *The ovum* (the fleshy substance) may be available to see.
b. *Vaginal bleeding* can be seen.
c. *Tenderness of the womb* can be elicited by pressing just above the pubic bone.

Actions

The mother must be taken to hospital because blood-loss can be very heavy. Preferably, contact her doctor who will arrange for her admission, but again, if you are out in the wilds, just get going. The best possible thing that you can do for the woman is to get her to hospital. You will do her not one scrap of good by keeping her away from hospital and the baby is doomed to die, anyway.

By now you should have a reasonable understanding of pregnancy and you should be able to understand that, if you find a pregnant woman who has been injured, then provided that:

1. There is no vaginal bleeding.
2. There is no abdominal pain.
3. There is no low backache.
4. There is no tenderness of the womb when you press around the abdomen.
5. The woman can feel movements (if she is far enough on in pregnancy).
6. The baby's heartbeat can still be heard (depending on the stage of pregnancy);
   then it follows that the pregnancy is still intact!

So there is no cause far alarm as far as the pregnancy is concerned.

It is important to reassure the woman about this *forthwith*.

15

The search for injuries in the unconscious patient

'How can I examine an unconscious person for injuries?' This is a very relevant and important question indeed, because ALL unconscious patients should be examined for possible injuries. Just as it is important to search for the non-obvious injuries in the conscious patient, it is even more important to search for injuries which may be present but which may not be obvious in the unconscious patient, *even if the cause of unconsciousness seems to be obvious*. A person who is known to be a diabetic, may be found lying unconscious and displaying the signs of hypoglycaemic (insulin) coma. The diagnosis may appear to be obvious and, of course, the priority is to treat the coma. Nevertheless, that person may have sustained an injury when falling. There is an old saying that a drunken man never hurts himself when he falls because he is very relaxed. This old saying is, in fact, absolute nonsense. A drunken man very often hurts himself when he falls, because his reactions are too slow and his co-ordination is too poor to protect him from injury. Therefore, although the cause of unconsciousness may be reasonably obvious, it is still important to search for possible injuries so that one can satisfy one's self as to the presence, or absence, of injuries.

When examining the unconscious patient, we must look for evidence of injury—i.e. lacerations, abrasions, bruising, oedema, fractures (not forgetting the 'give-away' signs described in 'Injuries to bones and joints) and evidence of chest or abdominal injury. During the examination, the following points should be borne in mind:

a. Shock (the signs of which are pallor, a cold clammy skin and a rapid thready pulse) is NOT a usual feature of head injury. Therefore,

(i) If the signs of shock are found in the victim of a head injury, look for an obvious cause—e.g. multiple fractures or a stove-in chest.

(ii) If the signs of shock are present and there is no obvious cause

206

such as multiple fractures or heavy external bleeding, then suspect internal injury or disorder—e.g. ruptured spleen, myocardinal in farct, tension pneumothorax, etc.

b. *Oedema* often overlies the site of a fracture in a subcutaneous bone. This applies especially to fractures of the skull.

c. *Serious chest conditions* are diagnosed mainly from signs as apposed to symptoms (e.g. a sucking chest wound).

d. *Visible bruising* on the abdominal wall usually indicates an internal injury. Other signs of abdominal injury may be absent, depending upon the depth of unconsciousness.

e. *The cardinal signs of fracture* are not all applicable in the unconscious person. Loss of function cannot be assessed properly in the unconscious, and localised bony tenderness is applicable only in someone who is in the equivalent of Stage 2 anaesthesia (the stage of subconscious excitement) because that person still responds to severely painful stimuli. However, a person who is in the equivalent of Stage 3 (i) anaesthesia (the stage of light surgical anaesthesia), or deeper, does not respond at all to very painful stimuli. Therefore, from this level of consciousness downwards, the only reliable cardinal signs of fracture are deformity, abnormal mobility, bony crepitus and the 'give-away' signs (e.g. the flattened deltoid muscle of a dislocated shoulder, or the attitude of the lower limb with the fractured neck of femur).

f. *The recovery position* need not always be adopted for a person in the equivalent of Stage 2 anaesthesia, since the basic reflexes of coughing, swallowing and 'gagging' are still functional. Therefore, that person can still protect his own airway. However, if such a person is having difficulty because of bleeding from a wound inside the mouth, then obviously the recovery position will ease the problem. At deeper levels of consciousness where the cough, swallow and 'gag' reflexes do not function, the recovery position is virtually mandatory unless the airway has been protected by the insertion of an endotracheal tube.

g. *The check for spinal injury*, particularly injury to the cervical spine (neck bones), should ideally be performed BEFORE moving the patient. This is a good, sound rule whether the patient is conscious or unconscious, because if a spinal injury (especially an injury of the neck) is found, it must be immobilised to prevent further damage.

The exceptions to the rule are:

(i) When an unconscious person vomits whilst lying on his back, thereby endangering his own airway, or if the integrity of his airway is at risk because of other reasons (e.g. heavy bleeding from inside the mouth). In such circumstances, he *must* be rolled *quickly* into the recovery position or he will asphyxiate and die. The integrity of the airway takes priority and, therefore, the risk of *possible* further damage to a *possible* spinal injury (*which may not exist, anyway!*) is an acceptable risk under such circumstances. I would also point out that, whilst rolling the unconscious patient into the recovery position, the neck should, as far as is possible, be protected from undue movement. Therefore, the manoeuvre is best performed by two people, one of whom protects the neck whilst the other rolls the patient over. If there is no second person, the lone first aider must turn the patient over quickly and hope for the best. It is also worth remembering that most spinal injuries are stable and that, in the case of the unstable spinal fracture, any damage to the spinal cord has probably been done already. Movement may aggravate this damage, but this risk must be accepted if the recovery position becomes mandatory or the patient will die.

(ii) When there is imminent danger from external sources—e.g. fire, a rockfall, or a live, high-tension cable. If the source of danger cannot be eliminated without moving the patient (e.g. by switching off the source of electricity), then the patient *must* be removed from the source of danger. Again, this should be done as carefully as possible, but if there is only one first aider present, and if he and the unconscious person are about to be buried by a rockfall or engulfed by fire, the first aider has no option but to drag the unconscious person to a place of safety.

One way of doing this is to grab hold of the person's coat-collar on either side of the neck and pull. This raises the coat-collar sufficiently to offer some protection against undue extension of the neck, whilst the position of the rescuer's hands prevents undue lateral flexion and rotation of the neck. So, if someone says, 'Grab him by the scruff of the neck and get the hell out of there!' then this is the safest way to do it. Furthermore, using this method a person can drag someone of greater weight with relative ease. My wife and I have proved this by practical experiment and my wife's weight is only about 70 per cent of my weight. Let us now proceed with the examination of the unconscious patient.

Procedure

1. On approaching the unconscious person, look for clues (such as an empty bottle of sleeping tablets) and for any source of further

danger. Note if there is a telephone available so that help can be summoned, and whether other people are present who could be valuable as witnesses to the event, or who can be of assistance in any way. If possible, send someone to summon the ambulance *forthwith*.

2. Eliminate external sources of danger if possible, or, if this is not possible, remove the patient from the source of danger as described in (g) (ii), above.

3. If there is no external source of danger, move the patient as little as possible until spinal injury has been excluded, except when the airway is in danger as in (g) (i) above, when the recovery position *must* be used.

4. Ensure and maintain the integrity of the airway.

5. Stop gross bleeding.

6. Check that the heart is still beating.

7. Check the pulse for rate, rhythm and volume.

8. Note if the signs of shock are present.

N.B. (a) The hallmark of the good first aider is the ability to adapt rapidly to the situation as it presents itself. Therefore, procedures 4, 5, 6, 7 and 8 are not necessarily to be followed in that exact order. For instance, if the patient is obviously still breathing but there is gross external bleeding, the priority is to stop the bleeding; but, if the airway is obstructed, and if it is not easily cleared by extending the head, then the priority is to roll the patient into the recovery position quickly, otherwise he could suffocate whilst you are stopping the gross bleeding. If there is no gross external bleeding, then you can check the pulse for rhythm and volume whilst, at the same time, noting the facial appearance and whether the patient is breathing or not. The exact pulse rate can be counted later. So, circumstances will dictate the order of actions to be performed.

(b) So far, we have dealt with only the basics of first aid, often referred to as 'the ABCs of first aid'. Depending upon the findings so far, it may be necessary at this stage to delay the rest of the examination whilst resuscitative measure are undertaken, such as cardiopulmonary resuscitation, emergency tracheotomy, or cricothyrotomy, and commencing intravenous fluids.

9. Examine the head, as described in 'Head injuries', remembering to check the pupils for size, equality, reaction to light and the consensual light reflex.

10. Examine the rest of the body as described in Part 11 ('The search for injuries'), bearing in mind the points mentioned above

in the preliminary paragraphs of this topic and points (a) to (g) above.

(*N.B.* At this stage, a doctor would administer whatever drugs were necessary.)

11. Perform whatever splinting and bandaging is necessary as quickly and efficiently as possible.

12. Ensure that the patient is in the appropriate position for transportation to hospital (e.g. lying on the right side if there is a right-sided stove-in chest injury).

13. Record the patient's vital signs (pulse, blood pressure, respiration, etc.), together with the findings and the treatment given.

14. Commence observation, as described in 'Head injuries', and record the observations regularly.

15. Get the patient to hospital as quickly as possible, but bearing in mind the comfort of the patient during the journey. A rough journey will aggravate shock, even in the unconscious patient!

16. On reaching hospital, hand over the patient and your records to the appropriate personnel. DO NOT leave the hospital immediately because the doctors and nurses may wish to question you.

17. Members of mountain rescue and cave rescue teams should ask the hospital personnal: (a) to return their records when they have obtained whatever information they require from them, so that an accurate report can be sent to the Mountain Rescue Committee which records all mountain and cave incidents, and (b) to return their equipment, because mountain and cave rescue equipment is too expensive *not* to reclaim!

16

Mass casualties

It does not take much imagination to realise that disasters can occur anywhere and at any time. The police have the ultimate responsibility for dealing with disasters and each police force already has contingency plans for dealing with disasters in its own area. Even when only one person is lost or injured, the police accept responsibility for the search for and the rescue of that person, even though the actual search and rescue may be carried out by a civilian search and rescue team. If follows, therefore, that if a person is lost or injured, or if mass casualties have occurred, the police *must* be informed without delay, because the police are in the best position to contact rescue teams, ambulance chiefs, fire brigade chiefs and hospitals.

The search for survivors in out-of-the-way places and the evacuation of those survivors should be conducted under the guidance of the most experienced mountaineer, fell-walker, potholer, etc. He is usually the Team Leader, anyway. Once the scene of the accident is reached, the most experienced First Aider should be given a free hand, and he may not be the Team Leader. The most experienced First Aider is the one who is the best at diagnosis, and he should be given a title to denote this. Let us call him the Chief First Aider. The Chief First Aider should have a group of trusted First Aiders to whom he can delegate duties and he should be well aware of the individual capabilities of each one of his First Aiders. The first thing to do is to clear the accident site as much as possible by telling two or three of his First Aiders to usher the walking casualties to one side. These First Aiders will then have the duty of going over all of the walking casualties from head-to-toe, recording names, ages, addresses, religion, next-of-kin, and any injuries found, as well as making sure that each casualty has no internal injury before he is finally and confidently declared to be a walking casualty. The exclusion of internal injury in someone who was walking when found is an important job and if one of the First Aiders suspects

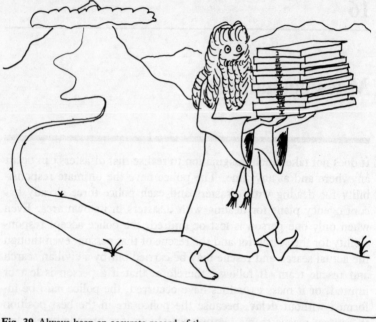

Fig. 39 Always keep an accurate record of the case.

an internal injury, he should report his suspicion to the Chief First Aider, who can then check the findings.

Whilst the walking casualties are being checked over systematically, the Chief First Aider and the rest of the First Aiders should go to work on the non-walking casualties. A useful time-saving measure would be for each First Aider to have with him another member of the team, *who can write legibly*, so that he can act as a clerk to the First Aider recording name, age, etc., and any injuries found, which would be dictated to him by the First Aider. By this method, a lot of people can be examined from head-to-toe and have their injuries recorded in a relatively short space of time. I stress again the importance of head-to-toe examination of every casualty *before* he is evacuated from the accident site. A suggested casualty record card is shown on page 215.

The Chief First Aider should soon be in possession of a list of injuries for each person. He can then check quickly for himself those who have the worst injuries and, having done so, the Chief First Aider must decide on his priority of evacuation. It is his duty, his decision and his responsibility alone. He is the one who is at the scene of the accident and who can see for himself the state of the injured people.

In fact, his duty involves him in the onerous task of *Triage*, which is the system whereby the injured are divided into three groups, A, B and C, as follows:

Group A consists of those, who are badly injured but recoverable and, therefore, in need of the most urgent treatment.

Group B consists of those who are injured, but whose injuries do not require urgent treatment.

Group C consists of the dead and the dying, i.e. those who are so badly injured that they are destined to die and are, therefore, irrecoverable (e.g. a man who is still just about breathing, but who has had half of his head blown away, is not going to survive much longer).

Groups A, B and C are evacuated in that order. Group C is last in the order of priority, because to evacuate someone from Group C in preference to someone from Group A, would waste valuable time, which could result in unnecessary loss of life in Group A.

If there is only one stretcher available, he must decide on the one person who needs to be given priority of evacuation, and this may be very difficult indeed. The Chief First Aider must make that decision and make it quickly, otherwise the rescue operation will be held up. When the decision has been made then it stands, whether it is right or wrong. Let there be no dissension in the ranks! If there is dissent, the rescue operation will assume a negative attitude; but if the Chief First Aider's decisions are arrived at quickly and adhered to, then the stretcher parties can get on with their job and the attitude of the whole rescue team will remain positive.

If there are (e.g.) three stretches available immediately, then the burden on the Chief First Aider is eased somewhat, because he can decide which three people are the most badly injured without having to decide which of these three people is in the worst condition. He simply tells the Team Leader who those three people are, and the Team Leader puts his stretcher parties to work. I shall return to the Chief First Aider's duties later.

The Team Leader is in overall command of his team during the rescue operation. There is no doubt about that! If the Team Leader gives an order, then all other team members *must obey*, because the Team Leader is responsible for the safety of his team. The Team Leader is also responsible for the evacuation of casualties and this poses the problem of evacuating the walking and the non-walking casualties. Obviously, when the non-walking casualties are ready the stretcher parties will waste no time in getting to work, because *speed of evacuation is vital*! This means that casualties should be transported as quickly *and as comfortably* as possible. If a person with a chest injury or an abdominal injury is transported rapidly and roughly, his general condition can deteriorate very quickly. This applies particularly to the mountain rescue situation, where speed of evacuation, comfort and the casualty's general condition must all be carefully assessed, so that the casualty eventually arrives at hospital in the shortest possible time commensurate with the least possible deterioration in his general condition.

If the Team Leader waits until all the non-walking casualities have been evacuated before he starts to evacuate the walking casualties, he may find that by this time, some of the walking casualties have begun to suffer hypothermia and may need a stretcher after all. Not only is this bad for the casualties but it is rather fatiguing for the stretcher parties! Therefore, I would *suggest* that the Team Leader divides his team members into stretcher parties and escort groups.

When the first half dozen or so of the walking casualties have been checked over to ensure that they are fit to be evacuated on foot, then it would need only two team members to escort them to safety, one in the lead and one bringing up the rear. Two more members could escort the next half dozen walking casualties whilst the first two were returning to the accident site. Preferably, the Team Leader should choose one evacuation route for the stretchers and a different route for the walking casualties, but it does not really matter if they all use the same route, provided that the walking casualties do not impede the progress of the stretcher parties.

Having begun the evacuation of the casualties, let us now return to the duties of the Chief First Aider. He has already decided on (let us say) his first three priority casualties, because they are already being evacuated by the stretcher parties. At the time of departure of those first three casualties, he had probably decided who were the next three casualties on the priority list and the next three after them, etc. However, this should not be an inflexible decision, because by the time the stretcher parties return, the situation could have changed, since one person's general condition may have deteriorated more rapidly than expected in relation to the general conditions of the other casualties. This can happen because we are all individuals and not machines. Some people have a physical resilience which others do not, and so as individuals, we respond to injury each in our own individual way. For this reason the Chief

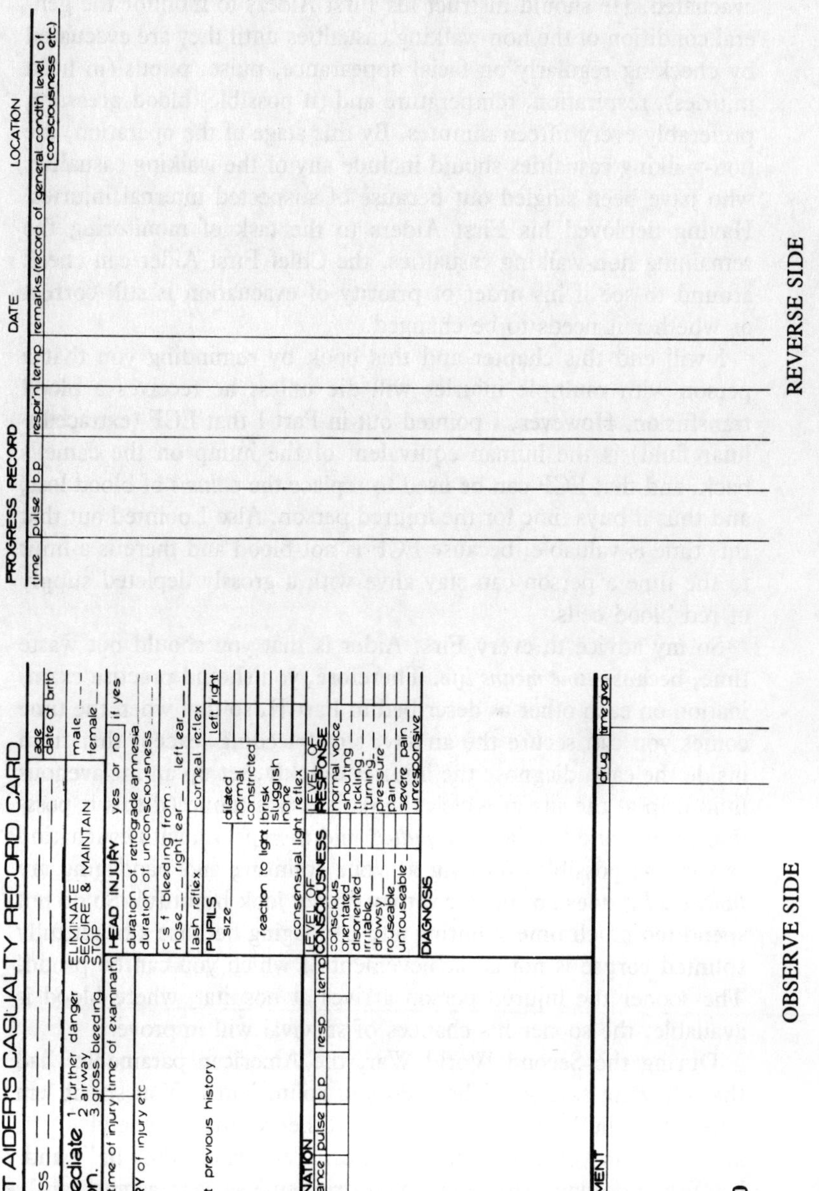

FIRST AIDER'S CASUALTY RECORD CARD

NAME _____
ADDRESS _____

age _____
date of birth _____

immediate action.
1 further danger
2 airway — ELIMINATE / SECURE & MAINTAIN
3 gross bleeding — STOP

male _____
female _____

date & time of injury / time of examination

HEAD INJURY — yes or no — if yes
duration of retrograde amnesia _____
duration of unconsciousness _____

HISTORY of injury etc

c.s.f bleeding from:
nose _____ right ear _____ left ear _____
lash reflex _____ corneal reflex _____

relevant previous history

PUPILS — left / right
size — dilated / normal / constricted
reaction to light — brisk / sluggish
consensual light reflex

LEVEL OF CONSCIOUSNESS
conscious
orientated
disoriented
irritable
drowsy
rouseable
unrouseable
unuseable

LEVEL OF RESPONSE
normal voice
shouting
ticking
turning
pressure
pain
severe pain
unresponsive

DIAGNOSIS

EXAMINATION
appearance	pulse	b.p	resp	temp

drug _____ time given _____

TREATMENT

OBSERVE SIDE

PROGRESS RECORD
time	pulse	b.p	respⁿ	temp	remarks (record of general condtn level of consciousness etc)	LOCATION

DATE _____

REVERSE SIDE

Fig. 40

First Aider cannot afford to relax until all the casualties have been evacuated. He should instruct his First Aiders to monitor the general condition of the non-walking casualties until they are evacuated by checking regularly on facial appearance, pulse, pupils (in head injuries), respiration, temperature and (if possible) blood pressure, preferably every fifteen minutes. By this stage of the operation, the non-walking casualties should include any of the walking casualties who have been singled out because of suspected internal injuries. Having deployed his First Aiders to the task of monitoring the remaining non-walking casualties, the Chief First Aider can check around to see if his order of priority of evacuation is still correct or whether it needs to be changed.

I will end this chapter and this book by reminding you that a person with multiple injuries will die unless he receives a blood transfusion. However, I pointed out in Part I that ECF (extracellular fluid) is the human equivalent of the hump on the camel's back, and that ECF can be used to replace the *volume* of blood lost, and thus it buys time for the injured person. Also I pointed out that this time is valuable, because ECF is not blood and there is a limit to the time a person can stay alive with a grossly depleted supply of red blood cells.

So my advice to every First Aider is that you should not waste time, because *time means life*. Therefore, you should practise examination on each other as described in Part II, so that when the time comes you can secure the airway, stop bleeding (except that from inside the ear), diagnose the injuries quickly, set up an intravenous fluid drip at the site at which the patient was found (if this is possible), splint and bandage *adequately* and then get on with evacuation as soon as possible. As long as your splinting and bandaging are *functional* it does not matter if they do not look beautiful. So do not spend too much time splinting and bandaging because a beautifully splinted corpse is not an achievement of which you can be proud! The sooner the injured person arrives at hospital, where blood is available, the sooner his chances of survival will improve.

During the Second World War, the American paramedics had the following saying: 'Where do you splint 'em?—You splint 'em where they lie!' They now have two other sayings, namely!
a. 'Where do you drip 'em?—You drip 'em where they lie!', and
b. 'When do you drip 'em?—You drip 'em? as soon as you can!'

Glossary

Air hunger. This is deep, sighing respiration. It is caused by gross loss of red blood cells.

Amnesia. This is loss of memory (i.e. inability to recall facts or events).

    a. *Anterograde amnesia* is loss of memory for events after a head injury (i.e. going forward in time from the time of the injury). It includes any period of unconsciousness.

    b. *Retrograde amnesia* is loss of memory for events prior to a head injury. The duration of retrograde amnesia is *directly* proportional to the severity of the head injury.

Anaphylaxis. This is an extremely severe hypersensitivity response to a foreign substance (e.g. penicillin, snake venom).

Apnoea. This means that a person is not breathing.

Apoplexy. This is commonly called a 'Stroke'. It is sometimes referred to as a cerebrovascular accident, or CVA for brevity. Examples are cerebral haemorrhage, cerebral thrombosis and subarachnoid haemorrhage.

Asphyxia. This is a condition in which the blood is grossly under-oxygenated. Its causes may be either physical or chemical. If the cause is not eliminated quickly enough, the victim of asphyxia will die.

Automatism. This is a condition, which may occur after an epileptic fit, and which may last up to twenty-four hours. It is characterised by the performance of routine, or automatic, actions, e.g. going for a bus ride on a certain bus route, or going to a certain cinema, or going for a walk on a specific route. In other words, these automatic actions have a define pattern.

Braxton-Hicks contractions. These are *painless* contractions of the womb, which occur during the last twelve weeks of pregnancy. They indicate that the womb is toning itself up for labour.

Cheyne-Stokes respiration. This is a form of respiration characterised by 'crescendos' of breathing interspersed with periods of apnoea (no breathing). It should *not* be confused with high-altitude respiration.

Compression of the brain. This is a condition caused by continuous bleeding inside the skull. The bleeding forms an ever-enlarging pool of blood within the skull. In turn, this ever-enlarging pool of blood exerts a continuous and ever-increasing pressure on the brain, inside the skull. Thus, the brain is gradually *compressed* by the enlarging pool of blood, within an inexpandible bony box (the skull). This condition should *not* be confused with a *depressed* skull fracture.

Concussion. This simply means brain damage. It is diagnosed from the history of a head injury, which has resulted in *retrograde* amnesia.

CSF. This is an abbreviation for cerebrospinal fluid. It is a crystal-clear fluid, which bathes the central nervous system (the brain and spinal cord). It lies between the brain and spinal cord, on the one hand, and their coverings (the meninges) on the other.

Diastole. This is the period during which the heart relaxes.

217

Dislocation. This is defined as 'complete loss of apposition of the surfaces of a joint'.

ECF. This is extracellular fluid. Strictly speaking it includes blood, CSF, the interstitial fluid and lymph—i.e. all the body fluids, which are *outside* the cells of the body. *For the purposes of the text of this book only*, ECF refers to the interstitial fluid—i.e. the fluid which lies between the bloodstream and the cells.

Effusion. This is an excessive amount of synovial fluid, or blood, or both, within a synovial joint. Usually, an effusion occurs as a result of injury. Sometimes, an effusion may be caused by disease or infection. In the case of infection, the effusion is quite likely to contain pus.

Embolism. This is the blocking of a blood vessel by a sufficiently large particle (or *embolus*) carried along by the bloodsteam. Embolism commonly causes *infarction* (i.e. death) of the tissues supplied by the blocked blood-vessel, e.g. myocardial infarction is the death of part of the heart muscle (or myocardium).

Embolus. This is the particle which causes an embolism. It may be (a) a detached blood clot, (b) detached, infected 'vegetations', from a diseased heart valve, (c) a fat embolus, which can occur after multiple fractures, or after the fracture of a large bone, or (d) an air embolus, which may occur accidentally, during an intravenous infusion of fluid, or during a blood transfusion. The commonest form of embolus is a detached blood clot.

Excretion. This is the process, by which unwanted by-products of metabolism are removed from the body.

Flail segment. See 'paradoxical respiration' below.

Haematoma. This is a collection of blood in an unusual position within the body, but outside the bloodstream. It usually occurs as a result of injury, but can occur spontaneously in certain diseases (e.g. Leukaemia).

Haemothorax. This is a collection of blood within the chest, or thorax. In effect, it is a haematoma inside the chest. The collection of blood lies between the lung and the chest wall. It is usually the result of an injury to the chest.

ICF. This is intracellular fluid—i.e. the fluid inside the body cells.

Infarct. *see* **Embolism.**

Liquor. (Pronounced, 'Lie-kwor'). This is a crystal-clear, rather sweet-smelling liquid. It bathes and protects an unborn baby inside the sac of membranes within the womb. This liquor should not be confused with alcoholic liquor (pronounced, 'Likkor').

Meninges. These are the coverings of the central nervous system (the brain and spinal cord).

Meniscus. (plural = menisci). This is a new-moon-shaped structure. There are two in each knee joint and their function is to facilitate rotational movements in the flexed, or semi-flexed, knee joint. They are commonly referred to as 'cartilages'. The TM joints also have menisci, to facilitate lateral (sideways) movements of the lower jaw.

Metabolic rate. This is the *rate* at which energy is produced and used.

Metabolism. This word means the production and use of energy.

Midclavicular line. This is an imaginary line, drawn perpendicularly from the midpoint of the clavicle, on either side. Since this line usually passes through the nipple, it is often called the 'nipple line'.

Movements. These are fetal movements, i.e. the movements of an unborn baby inside the womb. The mother may start to feel them any time from the sixteenth week of pregnancy onwards.

Muscle-spasm. This occurs after injury, reflexly. It reduces movement at the site of injury, which, in turn, reduces pain. It is Nature's own built-in, self-splinting mechanism.

Myocardial infarct. This is the death of all, or part, of the heart muscle. (*see* **Embolism**).

Neck rigidity. This means that the neck cannot be flexed so that the chin touches the chest. It occurs typically in meningitis, encephalitis and subarachnoid haemorrhage.

Oedema. This is a localised, excessive collection of tissue fluid. The fluid is interspersed amongst the cells locally. Typically, a 'pitting', or 'pitmark', can be made in oedema by pressing with a finger for about five seconds. This 'pitting' distinguishes oedema from a haematoma, which does not 'pit'. Oedema commonly results from injury. It may occur in association with fractures, where the bone lies just under the skin (e.g. skull, clavicle, ulna and tibia). When oedema of the scalp occurs, after a head injury, it is virtually always diagnostic of a fracture of the skull and it marks the fracture site. Oedema may also occur (a) in the feet, ankles and legs of a person, who is suffering from congestive heart failure and (b) locally, at the site of an acute infection (e.g. a boil or an abscess).

Olecranon process. This is the upper end of the ulna. Together with the upper end of the radius and the lower end of the humerus, it forms the elbow joint.

Opiates. These are drugs derived from Opium, which comes from the opium poppy. Typical examples are Pethidine, Morphine, Papaveretum ('Omnopon') and Diamorphine ('Heroin').

Paradoxical respiration. A condition in which a flail segment of the chest wall moves inwards during inspiration, whilst the rest of the chest wall moves outwards, and vice versa, during expiration. It occurs after a series of ribs has been broken, each in two places, to produce the flail (i.e. unstable) segment of the chest wall.

Peritoneum. This is the inner lining of the abdomen. It is rather sensitive to irritation, pain, etc.

Reactive hyperaemia. This is an excessive dilation of the blood vessels of the skin. It occurs after a period of constriction of the blood vessels (e.g. in response to a very cold environment).

Retroperitoneal haematoma. (see 'Haematoma'). This is a haematoma, which lies behind the peritoneum (the inner lining of the abdomen), but in front of the muscles, which cover the front of the lumbar spine. It results from injury, and can account for between two and four pints of blood loss.

Rigidity. This is the term used to describe muscle-spasm in the abdomen. It may occur in response to injury, or to disease (e.g. acute appendicitis, or perforated duodenal ulcer).

Shock. This is a clinical condition, characterised by pallor, a cold, clammy skin and a rapid, thready pulse. These three signs are always associated with a lowered blood pressure. (for types of shock, see text, p. 32).

Show. This is a blood-stained, mucus plug, which is released from the neck of the womb, either prior to labour, or during the first stage of labour.

Sign. This is something, which is found on examination of a person.

Situs inversus. This is a condition in which the apex beat of the heart is to be found in the right side of the chest, instead of in the left side of the chest, as in normal people. People, who have situs inversus, are usually quite healthy. In *complete situs inversus*, each organ is to be found in the opposite side of the body to that in which it is normally found (e.g. spleen on the right, appendix on the left). In fact, the whole of the body is a 'mirror image' of the normal arrangement of the human body.

Status epilepticus. This is a series of epileptic fits strung together—i.e. before one fit is completed, another fit begins, etc. If not treated promptly, it can be fatal.

Stroke. see **Apoplexy.**

Subluxation. This is defined as 'incomplete loss of apposition of the surfaces of a joint'.

Surgical emphysema. This is air in the soft tissues of the front of the neck. On palpation, it gives a soft, crinkly, tissue-paper-like feeling to the fingers. It results from a severe compression injury to the chest.

Symptom. This is something of which a patient complains, e.g. pain, inability to walk, etc.

Syncope. This is a sudden lapse into unconsciousness (i.e. a 'faint').

Synovial fluid. This is the fluid produced by the synovial membrane (the delicate inner lining) of a synovial joint. It lubricates the joint surfaces.

Systole. This is the period, during which the heart is contracting—i.e. pumping out blood.

Thrombosis. This is the formation of a blood clot, or thrombus. It usually occurs in a vein, but can occur in one of the coronary arteries, which supply the heart muscle, in which case a coronary thrombosis, or myocardial infarct, occurs, (*see* **Infarct**).

Uraemia. This is a condition, in which there is a gross build-up of urea and ammonia in the blood. It is indicative of serious kidney disease.

Urea. This is a harmless by-product of protein breakdown. Urea is excreted by the kidneys.

Uterus. This organ is commonly referred to as the womb. It serves as an incubator and as protection for an unborn baby during pregnancy, and its muscle provides the expulsive force required during labour.

Zygomatic arch. This is the bony arch, which can be felt, as it passes from the cheek-bone to just in front of the ear. There is one arch on each side of the face. These arches help to preserve the normal facial contours.

Index